ILLUSTRATED
MOXIBUSTION
THERAPY

Copyright © 2018 Shanghai Press and Publishing Development Co., Ltd.
Chinese edition © 2012 Chemical Industry Press

This book is edited and designed by the Editorial Committee of *Cultural China* series.

Text by Duan Xuezhong
Translation by Cao Jianxin
Design by Wang Wei

Copy Editor: Gretchen Zampogna
Editors: Wu Yuezhou, Cao Yue
Editorial Director: Zhang Yicong

Senior Consultants: Sun Yong, Wu Ying, Yang Xinci
Managing Director and Publisher: Wang Youbu

ISBN: 978-1-60220-037-1

Address any comments about *Illustrated Moxibustion Therapy: A Natural Way of Prevention and Treatment through Traditional Chinese Medicine* to:

Better Link Press
99 Park Ave
New York, NY 10016
USA

or

Shanghai Press and Publishing Development Co., Ltd.
F 7 Donghu Road, Shanghai, China (200031)
Email: comments_betterlinkpress@hotmail.com

Printed in China by Shenzhen Donnelley Printing Co., Ltd.
1 3 5 7 9 10 8 6 4 2

The material in this book is provided for informational purposes only and is not intended as medical advice. The information contained in this book should not be used to diagnose or treat any illness, disorder, disease or health problem. Always consult your physician or health care provider before beginning any treatment of any illness, disorder or injury. Use of this book, advice, and information contained in this book is at the sole choice and risk of the reader.

Quanjing provides the image on page 60.

ILLUSTRATED MOXIBUSTION THERAPY

A Natural Way of Prevention and Treatment through
Traditional Chinese Medicine

By Duan Xuezhong

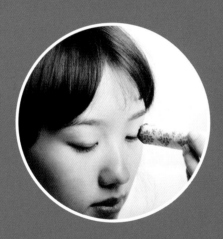

Better Link Press

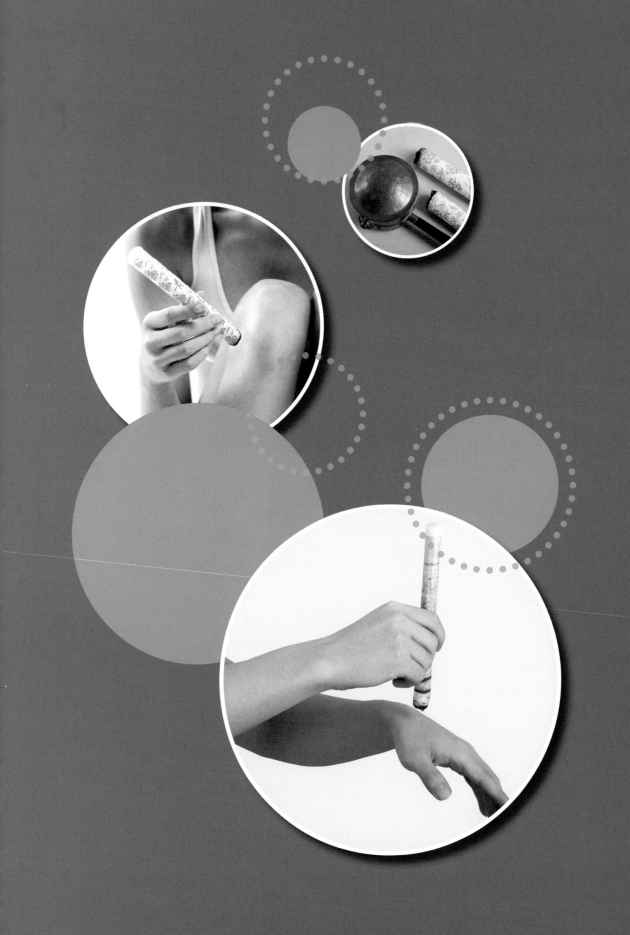

Contents

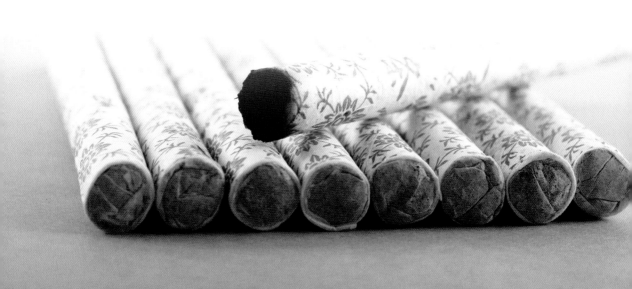

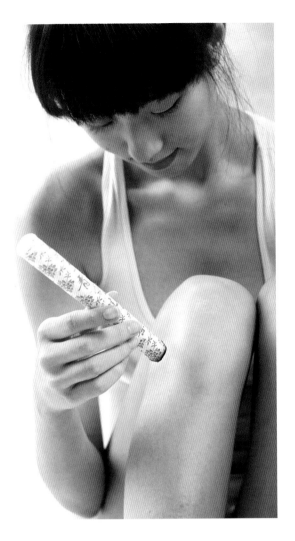

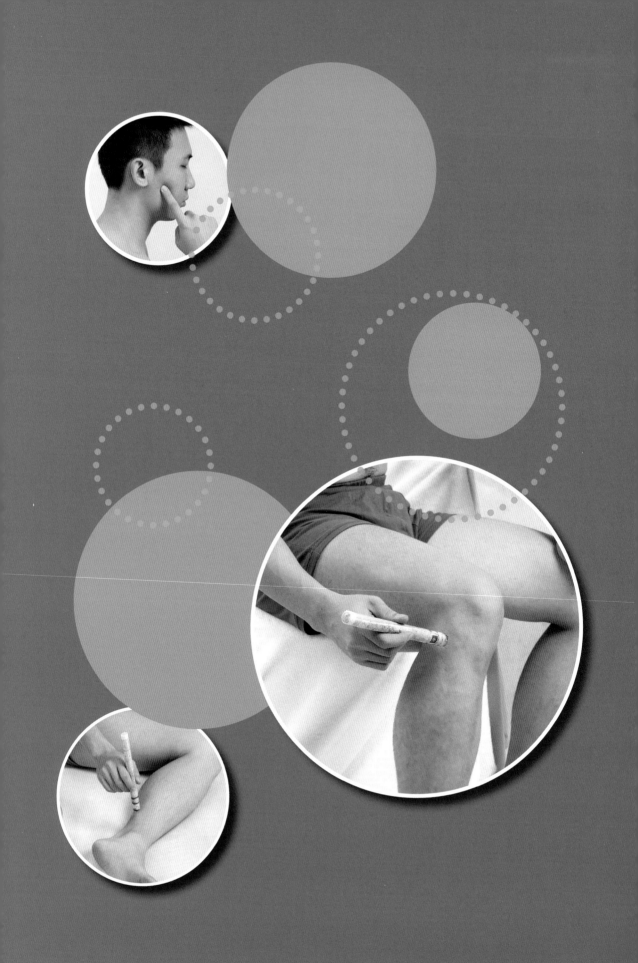

PREFACE

As living standards improve, we face ever-increasing pressure in our lives. Excessive fatigue and psychological burdens threaten our health, and various diseases cause decline in physical functions, which can lower our quality of life. Medical treatments and adverse reactions to medicines also bother people from time to time. Is there a way to enhance physical health and treat diseases without administering injections or taking medicine? This book introduces moxibustion as a natural therapy.

Moxibustion has been in use in China for thousands of years. People began using moxibustion extensively as early as in the Spring and Autumn Period and the Warring States Period (770 B.C. to 221 B.C.). The *Zhuangzi* wrote "Yue people smoked the affected area with moxa," and the *Mencius* also wrote that "treating a disease of seven years requires moxa aged for three years." There is a wide range of records about moxibustion in medical literature since ancient times, and the attraction of moxibustion hasn't dissipated over the generations.

Moxibustion is a therapy that involves burning loose moxa wool and moxa rolls made from mugwort leaves to target acupoints on the body. This thermal stimulation activates the meridians to help patients achieve health. This not only improves the circulation of qi (vitality) and blood, dredges meridians, regulates organ function and improves poor health, but can also relieve a variety of symptoms. The treatment is suitable for conditions related to internal medicine, surgery, gynecology and so on. Moxibustion is simple to practice, and even people with no medical knowledge can perform the therapy after some basic education. There are several methods of moxibustion. This book provides you with the safest and most effective procedures to keep you comfortable and healthy.

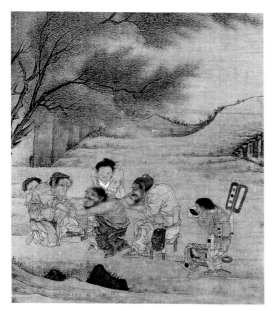

Moxibustion in ancient China.

This book consists of three parts. The first part gives a summary of moxibustion and introduces the concepts, benefits and materials of moxibustion, while presenting comprehensive knowledge of the therapy. The second part introduces the methods and techniques of moxibustion, describing commonly used methods, operation techniques, and points of attention in the process of moxibustion, guiding you through the steps. The third part introduces the moxibustion therapy for treating more than 100 common diseases. It contains detailed text descriptions, as well as vivid and lively real-life demonstration pictures so readers can practice easily.

I sincerely hope that this book will prove convenient and bring you health and happiness.

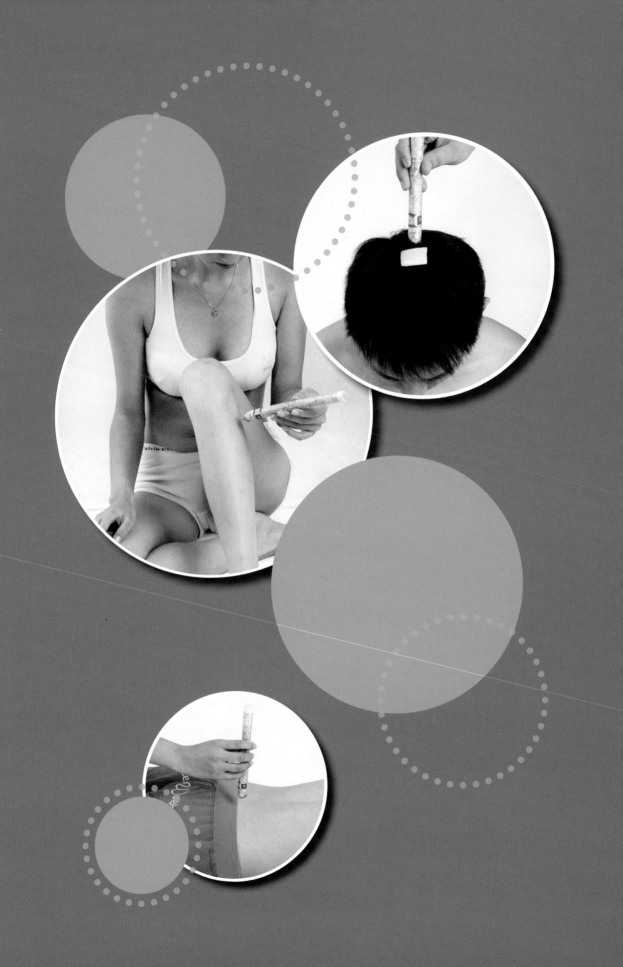

CHAPTER ONE
Introduction

Moxibustion therapy effectively warms yang and nourishes qi, dissolves stasis, and warms and dredges meridians through stimulating warmth applied to the skin. Simple to perform, moxibustion is a treasure of the traditional Chinese medicinal culture and one of the most ancient medical healthcare methods in traditional Chinese medicine (TCM). What is moxibustion, what benefits can moxibustion offer, and what needs to be prepared before moxibustion? This chapter will introduce the basic ideas of this treatment.

1. Concept

As the main disease treatment in ancient China, moxibustion was extensively popular in the Spring and Autumn Period and the Warring States Period. Because moxibustion therapy is simple, safe and effective, people without any medical knowledge can quickly grasp its methods with basic education. This quality has made moxibustion popular since ancient times. As a saying goes, "With moxa aged for three years, doctors go away."

Moxibustion therapy is a TCM therapy that involves burning loose moxa wool (P 12) to heat the acupoints on the human body. Moxibustion has a wide range of applications in internal medicine, surgery, gynecology, dermatology, ENT and other areas. It's particularly effective on mastitis, prostatitis, periarthritis of the shoulder, pelvic infection, cervical spondylosis and diabetes. Moxibustion can warm yang and nourish qi, dissolve stasis, and warm and dredge meridians, offering improved health for the whole body. There is a saying in China that "all diseases will disappear if the Zusanli point is warmed with moxa." Applying moxa to the Zusanli, Zhongwan, Mingmen, Qihai and Guanyuan acupoints will nourish stomach, yang qi, and essence and blood, thus strengthening the body's resistance, preventing diseases and offering good health. In modern times, moxibustion has remained an important healthcare methods.

2. Benefits

The mystery of moxibustion first comes from the pharmacological effects of moxa leaves. Moxa leaves having a warm medicinal property produce smoke when burned. The moxa smoke, together with the heat produced by the moxa fire, can warm qi and blood, warm meridians, expel the cold, and warm yang. The moxa leaf oil in the moxa smoke has good inhibitory effects on staphylococcus albus, group A streptococci, neisseria and pneumococcus. The main components of moxa leaf oil have the effects of exciting the nerve centers, relieving heat, stopping bleeding and easing pain.

The mystery of moxibustion also comes from its warm stimulation. Targeted warmth can improve local blood circulation and lymphatic circulation, accelerate cell metabolism, relieve inflammation and repair damaged tissues, so that muscles, nerve functions and structures can return to normal. The human body is an organic whole, with many factors affecting each other. Moxibustion can stimulate the body to produce a series of reactions, creating a benign regulatory effect to help treat diseases.

Different patients have different feelings during moxibustion and effects vary. Moxibustion is a treatment that needs to work through the body's internal reactions. Therefore, moxibustion therapy should be applied flexibly according to patients' specific conditions.

3. Materials and Instruments

Moxibustion materials come from the leaves of the mugwort plant, which can be made into moxa and further processed into moxa rolls. Some auxiliary instruments are also used in the moxibustion process, including a moxa box, moxa stick roll holder and so on. Below are brief descriptions to these materials and tools.

Mugwort

As recorded in *Compendium of Materia Medica* (*Bencao Gangmu*): "Mugwort leaf, as a medicine, is warm in property, bitter in taste, nontoxic and pure yang, can dredge 12 meridians, with the effects of restoring yang, increasing qi and blood circulation, expelling the cold and dampness, stopping bleeding and preventing miscarriage. It is often used in acupuncture and moxibustion."

Mugwort is a perennial herb, a slightly shrub-like plant with a strong aroma. It is mainly distributed in eastern Asia, including the Korean peninsula, Japan, Mongolia, and Northeast China, North China, East China, South China, Southwest China, Shaanxi Province and Gansu Province of China. When the mugwort plants flower, in the fourth to fifth lunar month of each year, they are picked and dried in the sun or in the shade for future use.

There are two main kinds of mugwort: One is mugwort planted in Qichun County and the other is wild mugwort. Mugwort in Qichun mostly grows north of the Yangtze River in China, with wide and thick leaves and much hair, and can be used to produce high-quality moxa wool. Wild mugwort mostly grows south of the Yangtze River in China, with a hard, velvety texture and poorer fragrance than the mugwort of Qichun. Wild mugwort is of inferior quality.

Mugwort leaves are aromatic, spicy, slightly bitter, warm, and pure yang in property. Moxibustion with mugwort leaves has such effects as dredging meridians, expelling the cold, eliminating swelling and nourishing yang.

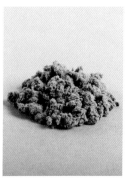

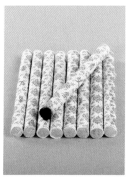

Loose moxa wool.   Moxa rolls.

Loose Moxa Wool

Thick, fresh mugwort leaves are picked in the fourth to fifth lunar month of each year, and repeatedly dried in the sun before being ground in a mortar and pestle or other device to a soft and cotton-like consistency. Stalks and dust are filtered out to yield thick moxa wool. To create thin moxa wool, the above steps are repeated, and the process yields clean, soft, thin yellow moxa wool.

The quality of moxa wool directly influences the effect of moxibustion. Good-quality moxa wool is free from impurities and is dry and soft with a fine velvety texture and can be stored for a long time. When it is burned, the fire is mild and not easy to disperse, and offers superior moxibustion effects. Poor-quality moxa wool generally contains more impurities and is damp and hard. It tends to burst when it is burned, making it easy to burn the skin. New moxa wool has strong fire and patients cannot always bear it.

Moxa Roll

A moxa roll is a cylindrical stick rolled with high-quality moxa wool, generally 20 centimeters long and 1.5 centimeters in diameter. If medicines are added into the moxa wool, the product is called a medicinal moxa roll and can be more effective than a regular roll. Patients can choose different moxa rolls according to their needs. Moxa rolls are available on Amazon and other online stores for convenient purchase.

Moxa Box

Moxibustion boxes come in different shapes, including cylindrical and conical. Most of the boxes have dozens of small holes at the bottom, and round holes on the wall. A small box is sheathed in the outer box for placing moxa wool and medicines. The outer tube has a handle for ease of use.

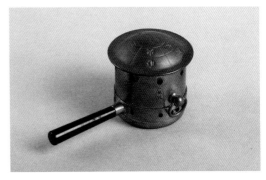

Moxa box.

To place moxa wool, first remove the inner box and put more than half a box of moxa wool or medicinal moxa wool inside. Gently press the moxa wool surface with your fingers—the moxa will not burn well if it's packed too firmly. Then place the small box into the outer box and ignite the moxa wool before replacing the top cover. Use several layers of cloth to cover the appropriate acupuncture point on the skin, and place the moxibustion box to the acupoint until local area of skin turns red and the patient feels comfortable. Moxibustion can last 15 to 30 minutes in general.

Moxa Stick Roll Holder

A moxibustion stick roll holder is a specially made wooden box-shaped moxibustion instrument, with one or more holes for placing moxa rolls. It is made of about half-centimeter-thick wood, without a bottom. On the top, there is a removable cover. A layer of wire gauze is placed in the box, 3 to 4 centimeters away from the bottom. There

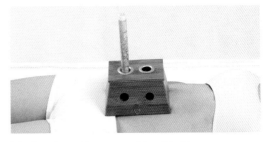

Moxibustion with a moxa stick roll holder.

are three sizes of moxibustion boxes—small, medium and large—and box size can be chosen based on the sizes of areas being operated on. To use the box, place the moxibustion stick roll holder onto the acupoint, and ignite a moxa roll and place it on the wire gauze before closing the cover. Apply moxibustion on the appropriate acupoint, generally for 15 to 30 minutes.

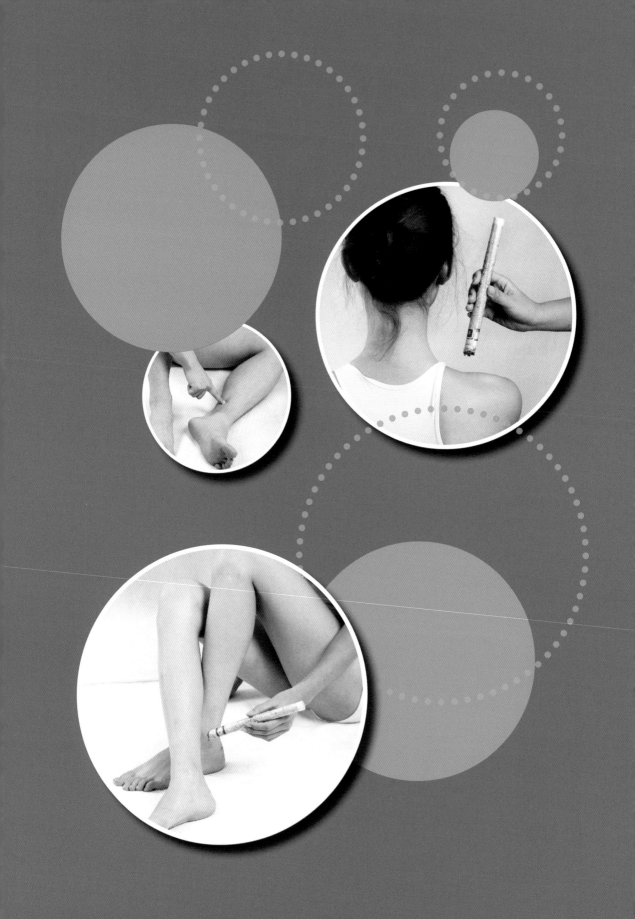

CHAPTER TWO
Methods and Techniques

The types and methods of moxibustion therapy have changed significantly over generations as physicians have accumulated experience. There are three commonly used methods of moxibustion, including moxibustion with a moxa cone, moxibustion with a moxa roll, and moxibustion with moxa smoke. We will focus on the latter two methods, which are popular in modern times for their safety and effectiveness.

The body position of patients, as well as quantity, order and time of moxibustion should be controlled, and desirable therapeutic effects on the diseases being treated can be achieved only by mastering these operation techniques and performing moxibustion accurately.

In addition, despite its wide application, moxibustion is banned from certain acupoints and there are some points of attention during the operation. These will also be introduced in this chapter.

1. Methods

The most frequently used methods of moxibustion are moxibustion with a moxa roll and moxibustion with moxa smoke. The first involves igniting a moxa roll at one end and placing it above an acupoint or an affected area. The most prevalent moxa roll method is over-skin moxibustion, which is further divided into mild moxibustion, swirling moxibustion and sparrow-pecking moxibustion. During practice, prevent moxa ash from falling to avoid burning the skin. Moxibustion with moxa smoke consists of three methods, including smoke moxibustion, steam moxibustion and moxibustion with a moxa burner.

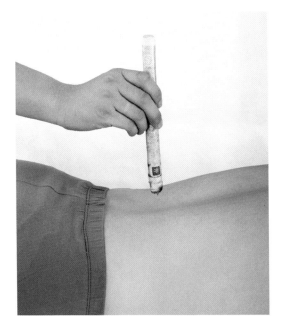

Mild moxibustion.

Mild Moxibustion

The ignited end of a moxa roll is pointed at the skin and kept 3 to 5 centimeters over a specific area, which allows the patient to feel warmth in the local area with no pain. Hold the roll for 20 minutes at each point until the skin reddens.

Characterized by constant and sustained temperature, this method can disperse local qi and blood stagnation, which is suitable for curing local diseases and pain. For a patient with reduced sensitivity, the practitioner should pay attention to feeling the temperature of the patient's skin to prevent burns.

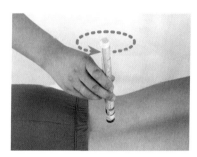

Swirling moxibustion.

Swirling Moxibustion

The ignited end of a moxa roll is pointed at the area for moxibustion, kept about 3 centimeters above the surface of the skin. Move the roll left and right or circularly, generally for 20 to 30 minutes.

This method is characterized by not only dispersing local qi and blood stagnation but also promoting the circulation of qi and blood in the meridians all over the body. Therefore, it has certain therapeutic effects on ailments in areas remote to the moxibustion points.

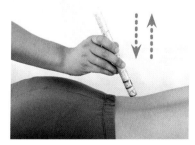

Sparrow-pecking moxibustion.

Sparrow-Pecking Moxibustion

Ignite a moxa roll at one end and move it up and down over the area for moxibustion, like a sparrow pecking at food, with the distance between the ignited end and the skin's surface kept between 2 and 3 centimeters. Generally, moxibustion lasts 5 to 15 minutes for each point.

This method is characterized by an alternating drop and rise in temperature, which can strongly arouse the functions of acupoints and meridians. Therefore, it is suitable for ailments and visceral diseases remote to the moxibustion points.

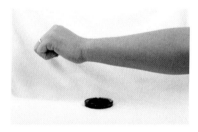

Smoke moxibustion.

Smoke Moxibustion

Burn moxa wool in an incombustible container and allow the skin's surface at the acupoints or affected areas to be exposed to the smoke. This method is suitable for joint pain caused by such pathogenic factors as wind, cold and dampness.

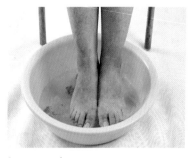

Steam moxibustion.

Steam Moxibustion

Boil mugwort leaves or moxa wool in water and allow the acupoints or affected areas to be exposed to the steam to cure arthralgia caused by such pathogenic factors as wind, cold and dampness.

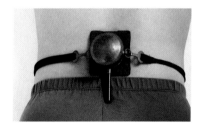

Moxibustion with moxa burner.

Moxibustion with Moxa Burner

Moxa burners usually include moxa box and moxa stick roll holder (P 13). Place moxa wool or a moxa roll in the burner and then put the burner on the acupoints for moxibustion. This method creates evenly distributed heat, which gives patients comfortable, warm stimulation and promotes qi and blood circulation. It is suitable for arthralgia caused by such pathogenic factors as wind, cold and dampness, stomachache and abdominal distension.

2. Operation Techniques

In performing moxibustion, first choose a correct body position to facilitate correct location of acupoints by the practitioner and make the patient feel comfortable. Be sure to maintain the posture throughout the entire process. Secondly, follow a certain moxibustion order, and determine the length of moxibustion time depending on the patient's specific conditions. During moxibustion, the patient can also judge the degree of relief from illness through body sensation, thereby determining the course of treatment. After moxibustion, pay attention to health care. Besides the techniques used for the moxibustion process, this chapter will also introduce to you the acupoints used for the therapy, the concept of acupoints and how to locate them quickly, making the moxibustion process simpler and more effective.

Body Position

Commonly used body positions include sitting and lying down. The sitting postures are divided into prone-supported sitting, lateral-supported sitting, and supine-supported sitting; the lying postures are divided into supine, prone and lateral postures.

Prone-supported sitting: The patient sits by a table on which a soft pillow is placed, and then the patient bends over the soft pillow or supports the forehead with both arms to expose the areas for moxibustion. This posture is suitable for the points on the back of head, neck and back, and sometimes for points on the forearms.

Lateral-supported sitting: The patient sits by a table on which a soft pillow is placed, and laterally bends over the table to expose the areas for moxibustion. This posture is mainly suitable for the points on both sides of the head.

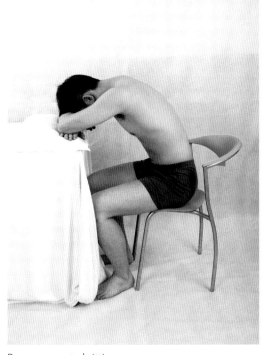

Prone-supported sitting.

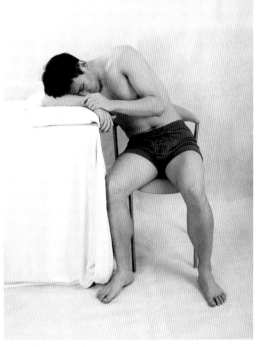

Lateral-supported sitting.

Supine-supported sitting: The patient sits in a supine position on a chair. This posture is mainly suitable for the treatment of such locations as the front of the head, cheeks, upper chest, shoulders, arms, legs, knees and ankles.

Lying on the back: The patient lies naturally on a bed in a supine position, with the arms placed on both sides of the body, the legs separated naturally, and the whole body relaxed with a soft pillow supporting the knees. This posture is suitable for the treatment of the head and face, chest, abdomen, inner side of the upper arms, the front, inside and outside of the legs.

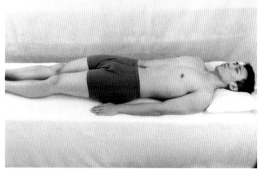

Lying on the back.

Lying prostrate: The patient lies naturally facedown in bed in a prone position, with one soft pillow placed before his chest and one underneath the ankles. This posture is suitable for the treatment of the neck, back, waist, buttocks and backs of both legs.

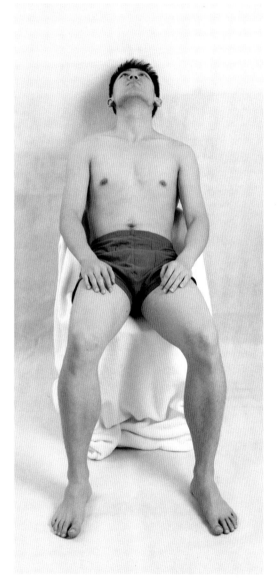

Supine-supported sitting.

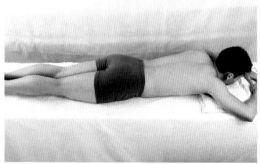

Lying prostrate.

Lying on the side: The patient lies on the side, with arms placed before the chest and the legs bent slightly. This posture is suitable for the treatment of the shoulders, ribs, hips, knees and outside of the arms and legs.

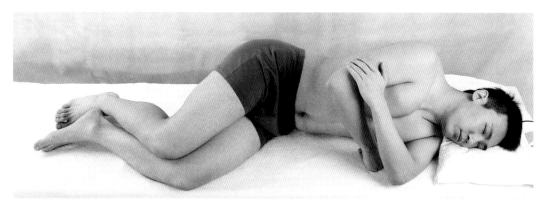

Lying on the side.

Order

In addition to a suitable body position, a certain order shall also be followed in the process of moxibustion to enhance the effect of the therapy. The usual order of performing moxibustion is upper body first, and then lower body; the head first and then the four limbs; the back first and then the chest and abdomen; yang channels first and then yin channels. However, when performing moxibustion, one ought to be flexible in selecting the order depending on different conditions.

Location

According to the theoretical system of Chinese medicine, main and collateral channels are regarded as the system linking the inside and outside of the human body as well as all inner organs. These channels run all through the body, connecting internal organs, limbs and joints, smoothing the circulation of vital energy and blood, and nurturing tendons and bones. Roughly speaking, there are 12 channels, including Taiyin Lung Meridian of Hand (LU), Jueyin Pericardium Meridian of Hand (PC), Shaoyin Heart Meridian of Hand (HT), Yangming Large Intestine Meridian of Hand (LI), Shaoyang Sanjiao Meridian of Hand (TE), Taiyang Small Intestine Meridian of Hand (SI), Yangming Stomach Meridian of Foot (ST), Shaoyang Gallbladder Meridian of Foot (GB), Taiyang Bladder Meridian of Foot (BL), Taiyin Spleen Meridian of Foot (SP), Jueyin Liver Meridian of Foot (LR), Shaoyin Kidney Meridian of Foot (KI) as well as Ren Meridian and Du Meridian.

Acupoints are special points on the body surface where the transport and transmission of vital energy and blood of human organs as well as main and collateral channels are concentrated. They are mostly distributed along the route of main and collateral channels as well as the places passed through by dense nerve endings or thick nerve fibers. Apart from those single points on the central axis of the human body, all the other acupoints are bilaterally symmetrical. These points are in close connection with the tissues and organs deep under the skin. Therefore, acupoints are reflecting points of diseases and stimulating points for treatment. There are also extra acupoints on the head and neck (EX-HN), on the chest and abdomen (EX-CA), on the back (EX-B), on the upper limbs (EX-UE) and on the lower limbs (EX-LE). Stimulation via moxibustuion at certain acupoints can effectively mobilize human ability to resist illness, preventing and curing illness.

The more accurately you find the location of the acupoint, the better the effects of the moxibustion will be. There are two methods of locating acupoints: Body length measurement and using fixed physical marks of the body.

Body Length Measurement

1. Use Thumb Length

The width of the patient's thumb joint is 1 cun. This is applicable for locating the acupoints on the arms and legs with vertical cun.

2. Use Middle-Finger Length

With the middle sections of the patient's bent middle finger as measurement, the distance between two inner crease tips is taken as 1 cun, which is mostly applicable for locating acupoints on the arms and legs with vertical cun and on the back with horizontal cun.

3. Use Four Fingers Closed Together

With the patient's index finger, middle finger, ring finger, and little finger stretched straight and closed, measure at the level of the large knuckle (the second joint) of the middle finger. The width of the four fingers is 3 cun.

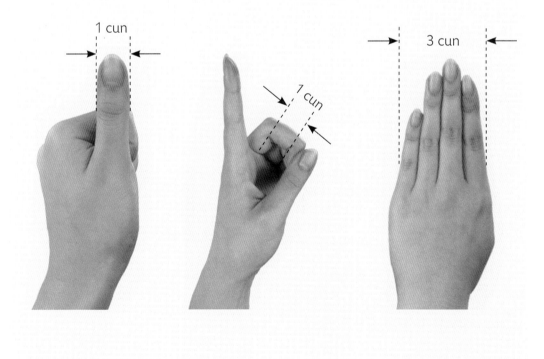

Physical Marks of the Body

1. Use Fixed Marks

These are fixed marks free from the movement of the human body, such as the mouth, ears, nose, eyes, hair, fingernails, toenails, breasts and navel, as well as various protruding bone joints and cavities. They are ideal for locating acupoints since they remain unmovable. For instance, the Yintang point lies between the two eyebrows, the Danzhong point lies between the two nipples, the Tianshu point is 2 cun away from the navel, and the Dazhui point lies under the seventh spinous process of the cervical spine when the patient lower the head.

2. Use Special Postures

This refers to the marks that only appear when corresponding movement takes place, including the appearance of the pores, cavities and wrinkles as the joints, skin and muscles move around, and sometimes the limb movement. For instance, the Tinggong point is in a cavity in front of the tragus when the one opens the mouth, and the Houxi point can be found at the end of the palm crease when one grips the fist.

3. Use Experience

This is a simple and convenient method accumulated through long-term practice. For instance, with the hand drooping vertically, the point touched by the tip of the middle finger is Fengshi point. With two hands crossed naturally and flatly between the thumb and the index finger, the point touched by the tip of the index finger is Lieque point.

Finding the most painful point is another method of locating acupoints, i.e., Ashi point. Acupoints of this sort are generally decided by the kind of diseases, mostly near the place with pathological change, or at a point quite far away from it. Ashi point has no fixed position or name. The place with pain is the location of the point, so it's commonly known as "wherever there is pain, there is an acupoint."

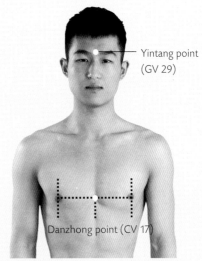

Yintang point (GV 29)

Danzhong point (CV 17)

Use fixed marks. Get Yintang point between the eyebrows and Danzhong point between the nipples.

Quantity of Moxibustion

This refers to the heat infused into the body during moxibustion therapy. It mainly depends on the length of treatment time, the area of moxibustion, and the degree of warmth during treatment. Different moxibustion quantities will produce different effects. The control of quantity affects the results of moxibustion, which seems simple, but only after longtime observation and accumulation of experience can one control it accurately and achieve the best therapeutic outcome.

The length of moxibustion time depends on such factors as physique, age, body regions, and the patient's condition. Chronic cases call for a long course of treatment and a large quantity of moxibustion, while acute cases require a shorter course of treatment and smaller moxibustion quantity.

The area of moxibustion and degree of warmth received during treatment will mainly depend on the size, number, and fire of moxa rolls, and the time duration of moxibustion with a moxa rolls or moxa burner. The moxibustion quantity will be large if the moxa rolls are large or numerous, the fire is strong, or the time duration of moxibustion is long. Otherwise, the moxibustion quantity is small.

Then how to control the moxibustion quantity? The following rules can be followed:

Duration: Moxibustion quantity will vary with different methods of moxibustion. Mild moxibustion (P 15) with a moxa roll (P 13) lasts 10 to 15 minutes each day, swirling moxibustion (P 16) lasts 20 to 30 minutes a day, and sparrow-pecking moxibustion (P 16) lasts 5 to 15 minutes a day. The duration of moxibustion with a moxa burner is relatively long, but should be less than 30 minutes, depending on the conditions and the patient's feelings during the therapy.

Times: In acute cases, perform treatment 2 to 3 times per day, while in chronic cases, perform one treatment once every 3 to 5 days. For general health care purposes, perform 3 to 4 times every month.

According to the physique: The moxibustion quantity can be large for a strong young male with a relatively good physique, but small for those who are weak, fatigued, old and for females.

Depending on the body parts: The moxibustion quantity can be large for muscular parts, such as the lower back, buttocks and abdomen. The moxibustion quantity should be small for the head, face, the hands and feet, and body parts with many veins or bones.

Depending on state of illness: The moxibustion quantity can be large for those with inveterate pathogenic cold (commonly seen in people with weak physique or hypofunction due to chronic disease), and for those whose vigor almost disappears, to replenish yang energy and expel cold. The moxibustion quantity should be small for patients with exogenous cold, to warm and activate meridians, and dispel exogenous pathogens.

The practitioner should flexibly control the moxibustion quantity during treatment, and not apply the rules mechanically. Factors like the nature and seriousness of illness, physique, age and different body parts should be considered.

Feelings during Moxibustion

During moxibustion, patients sometimes have sensations of heat, wind, cool, cold, numbness, bloating, soreness, sinking, pain and more. These feelings are the result of the joint efficacy of moxa's heat and medicine, and the manifestation of the fight between the circulating moxa fire and meridian qi and morbid qi. The sensations during moxibustion have a close relationship with therapeutic effects.

The feelings of moxibustion vary in each stage. There are three distinct stages in the moxibustion process. The first stage is characterized by the moxa fire flowing in the meridians. In this stage, the sensation is mild warmth, which is a benign reaction, and the patient feels comfortable with their ailment alleviated. The second stage is the fight between healthy and pathogenic factors. In this stage, sensations of numbness, bloating, soreness, sinking and pain can occur; these are normal reactions of the body. The third stage is when the body expels the pathogens. In this stage, feelings of wind, coolness and cold are normal reactions that result from the flow of pathogenic factors out of the body.

The feelings during moxibustion can be further categorized into seven different manifestations. The first is the heat penetrating directly from the skin's surface to deep tissues. The second is the heat diffusing from the moxibustion points to larger areas. The third is the heat moving from the moxibustion points to the remote areas via meridians, and even to the focus of the illness. The fourth is no heat in the moxibustion points, but heat in remote areas. The fifth is no heat on the skin's surface, while the deep skin or inner organs feel hot. The sixth is sensations of soreness, bloating, numbness, heat, sinking, pain, and cold in the skin or remote areas of the moxibustion points. The seventh is the deep and remote dispersion of the feelings from the moxibustion points, and easing of the symptoms. The sixth and seventh feelings of moxibustion mean the moxibustion has achieved the expected therapeutic effects.

The strength of the feelings during moxibustion represents the level of the meridians' blockage. Absence of sensation represents serious meridian blockage, which requires a long treatment time to dredge the meridians and eliminate stagnation, generally with slow effects. Strong feeling represents smooth meridians and good therapeutic effects. The person receiving moxibustion can judge the degree of recovery based on the feelings during moxibustion, to determine the course of treatment.

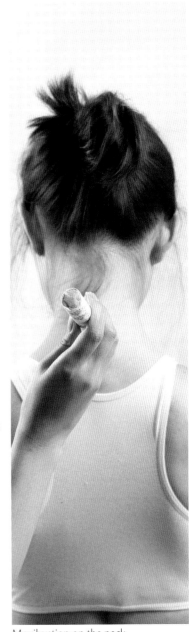

Moxibustion on the neck.

Health Care and Accident Treatment after Moxibustion

The post-moxibustion reactions differ from one person to another because of varying body tolerance, as well as different or inappropriate therapeutic methods. Ignore any red moxibustion marks with a scorched feeling, as they can disappear naturally. However, blisters and other wounded areas should be dealt with promptly. Attention should also be paid to post-moxibustion health care.

Vitality is expended during moxibustion for dredging meridians and regulating and replenishing body functions. Therefore, pay attention to protecting the body's vitality after moxibustion, using diet and other aspects of daily life to promote recuperation. Maintain a proper balance between work and rest, avoid fatigue and excessive activity, and keep a calm mood. Ensure sufficient sleep every day because sleep is the best way to recover strength. Do not eat raw, cold or indigestible food. Food should be light, with a vegetable diet and more fruits to supplement the nutrients required by the body.

Injuries caused by accidents during moxibustion must be dealt with promptly.

• **Treatment of Blisters**

Do not prick the blisters when they are small, and they should be absorbed naturally within about a week. If the blisters are big, it is advisable to first prick them with a sterile needle to discharge the liquid, then apply an anti-inflammatory cream before wrapping with a sterile gauze bandage. The gauze should be disinfected and replaced regularly to prevent infection.

• **Treatment of Moxibustion Sores**

If there is suppurative infection due to moxibustion sores, clean the sores with disinfectant, alcohol or normal saline. After that, take antibiotics orally and apply anti-inflammatory ointment. Continue to clean and apply the medicine until the sores are cured. Eat appropriate amount of foods that help remove pathogenic factors from the body, such as beans, mushrooms and bamboo shoots. When moxibustion sores begin to heal, reduce the intake of these foods, and keep the diet light; do not eat spicy or irritating food, and avoid heavy physical work. If moxibustion sores are infected, oral antibiotics and antiseptic ointment should be applied to promote wound healing.

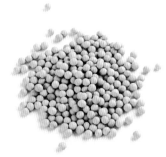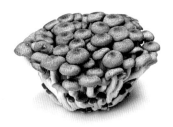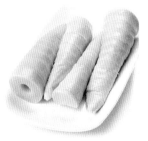

Beans, mushrooms and bamboo shoots.

3. Taboos and Points of Attention

Moxibustion can remove dampness, expel cold, regulate yin and yang, restore yang and rescue the patient from collapse, as well as prevent and cure diseases. Despite a wide range of applications, moxibustion cannot be applied to some parts of the body or some people, as essence and blood can be consumed during moxibustion. The taboos and points of attention should be followed strictly.

Taboos

Prohibited point: According to the modern traditional Chinese medicine, there is actually only one point contraindicated for moxibustion: the Jingming point (on the facing page).

Moxibustion should not be performed when a patient is excessively hungry, full, drunk, terrified, furious or thirsty.

Moxibustion should not be performed during the menstrual period.

Patients having dysphoria with feverish sensations in the chest, palms and soles, red face and ears, and internal accumulation of pathogenic heat should not receive moxibustion therapy.

Moxibustion should not be applied to the areas where the skin is thin or muscles are few, and the lumbosacral area and lower abdomen of pregnant women. It's also prohibited on nipples, private parts and testicles.

It also cannot be applied to the heart region or areas where big vessels are located.

Moxibustion should not be applied in the case of infectious diseases, high fever, coma, convulsions, or to patients who are in extreme exhaustion and thinned to the bone.

Mental patients should not receive moxibustion therapy.

Points of Attention

The practitioner should concentrate and perform all procedures with care. Be careful to avoid burning the skin with falling moxa ash and be sure to prevent the moxa roll from moving to an inappropriate point.

The points should be located accurately, and the body position should be comfortable. To ensure the effects of moxibustion therapy, consult a physician if you are unable to locate the points. The patient should choose a comfortable body position they can hold for the entire treatment.

Pay attention to the fire. After the completion of moxibustion, the fire should be extinguished to avoid a fire accident. When there is an excessive accumulation of moxa ash, blow it away before continuing treatment to avoid burning the skin or clothes with falling ash.

Pay attention to keeping warm or preventing heatstroke. Keep the patients warm during moxibustion in the winter to prevent catching a cold. In summer, the hot weather and the heat from moxa roll may cause heatstroke. Therefore, pay attention to adjusting the room temperature.

Do not perform moxibustion when the patient is hungry or immediately after a meal.

Prevent fainting from moxibustion. Do not panic if dizziness, blurred vision, nausea and other unpleasant phenomena occur during moxibustion. Stop moxibustion immediately, let the patient lie down and keep quiet, and then warm the Zusanli point for about 10 minutes with mild moxibustion.

Pay attention to adjusting the temperature of moxibustion. Feel the temperature of moxibustion area during the operation, especially for those who are slow in sensitivity, to prevent burning the skin with excessive heat.

Follow the principle of gradual and orderly progress. In the initial effort, use a small dose and a shorter time, and then gradually increase the dosage and extend the time, allowing the patient to acclimate to the therapy.

Pay attention to post-moxibustion health care. Patients should try to stay optimistic and happy, avoid heavy physical labor, and eat light and nutritious food. Throughout this

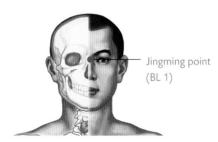

Jingming point
(BL 1)

book, the author has recommended many helpful recipes to the ailments, in which all figures in grams are converted into ounces, and the number is rounded to the nearest first decimal place for readers' convenience. You can be flexible in the amount of these ingredients to your taste.

Jingming point.

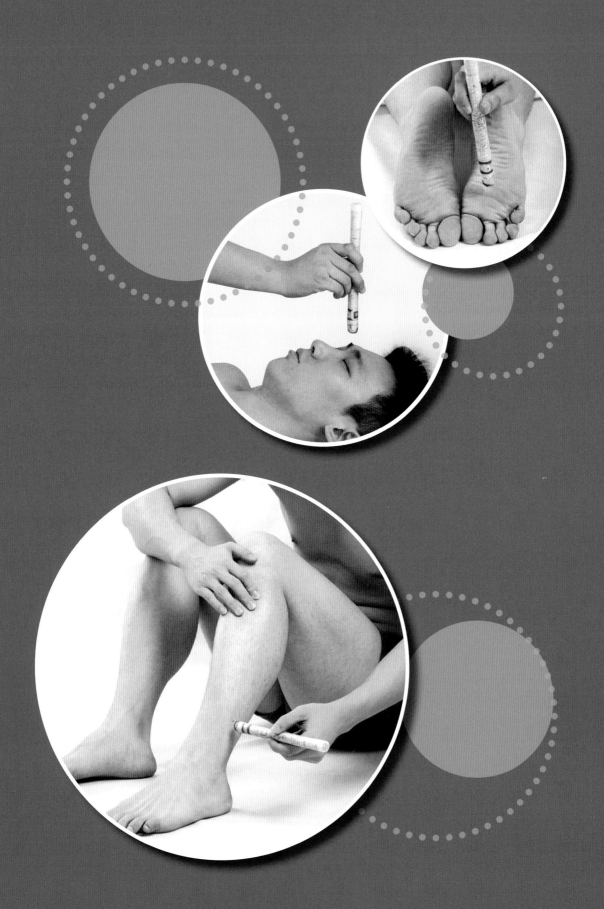

CHAPTER THREE
Moxibustion Therapy for Common Diseases

As a green therapy, moxibustion is pain-free and without side effects. It is so simple that people without even basic TCM knowledge can grasp it quickly. Moxibustion can offer not only general health care, but also cure many common diseases.

1. Cold

A cold is a self-healing disease, characterized by upper respiratory tract inflammation caused by viral or bacterial infection. Common symptoms are headache, fever, fatigue, cough, sneezing, sore throat and so on, and some patients also have digestive tract symptoms.

When suffering from a cold, you should eat light meals and avoid eating cold, greasy and spicy food. Also drink plenty of water as this is helpful for reducing fever, promoting sweating, and discharging toxins, and eat more vegetables and fruits rich in vitamins. During the cold, pay attention to striking a proper balance between work and rest, having more rest and less exercise, and taking fewer antibiotic drugs. Avoid crowded places where you could pass the disease to others.

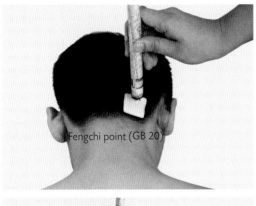

Fengchi point (GB 20)

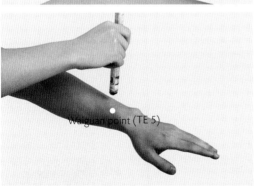

Waiguan point (TE 5)

Moxibustion Method

Mild moxibustion: Moxibustion is applied to the Fengchi, Dazhui, Quchi and Waiguan points, beginning with the head and then the four limbs. The practitioner, standing on one side of the patient who is sitting, lights one end of a moxa roll and directs the ignited roll head to an acupoint, 3 to 5 centimeters above the surface of the skin, until the skin feels warm without the feeling of burning pain.

Place a piece of ginger when applying moxibustion to the Fengchi point, so as not to ignite the hair. Moxibustion should last 3 to 5 minutes for each acupoint, until the patient has a warm feeling. If the patient is insensitive to the heat, the practitioner can place the index finger and middle finger on each side of the acupoint to feel the temperature and avoid burning the skin. Such treatment should be given once or twice per day; perform two more days after symptoms alleviate.

Acupoints of Moxibustion

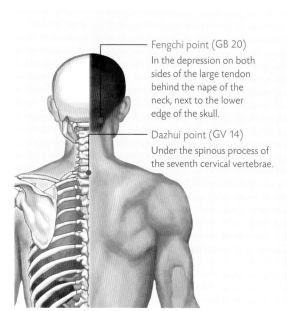

Fengchi point (GB 20)
In the depression on both sides of the large tendon behind the nape of the neck, next to the lower edge of the skull.

Dazhui point (GV 14)
Under the spinous process of the seventh cervical vertebrae.

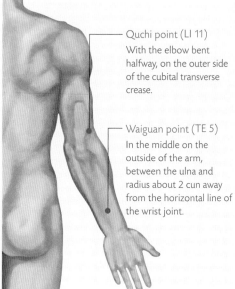

Quchi point (LI 11)
With the elbow bent halfway, on the outer side of the cubital transverse crease.

Waiguan point (TE 5)
In the middle on the outside of the arm, between the ulna and radius about 2 cun away from the horizontal line of the wrist joint.

1. Cabbage Soup with White Turnip
Ingredients: 17.6 ounces of Chinese cabbage heart, 4.2 ounces of white turnips, appropriate amount of brown sugar.
    Preparation: Mince the Chinese cabbage heart finely, cut the white turnips into thin slices, and add 27.3 ounces of water to cook. Add appropriate amount of brown sugar when 13.7 ounces of water are left. Then drink it. This receipt should be taken 6.8 ounces twice daily for consecutive 3 to 4 days. It serves to reinforce spleen functions, nourish lungs and warm up the body against the cold, and is suitable for dealing with the cold caused by pathogenic wind and heat.

2. Apple and Honey Water
Ingredients: Five apples, appropriate amount of lemon juice and honey.
    Preparation: Peel the apples, cut them into small pieces, add 34.2 ounces of water, boil for five minutes. After it is cooled to 104°F, add a small amount of lemon juice and appropriate amount of honey, and mix them. It should be taken several times a day in a small amount each time. Apple juice contains rich nutrients and it speeds up intestinal movement. Monosaccharide in the honey can be directly absorbed by the human body, which can promote the regeneration of liver cells and strengthen disease resistance.

2. Headache

Headaches are generally limited to pain in the upper half of the head, including the arch of the eyebrows, the upper edge of the helix and the areas above the external occipital protuberance. There are many causes for headaches, some of which are serious illnesses, but they are often difficult to pinpoint.

According to the traditional Chinese medicine, headaches are usually caused by wind-cold, wind-damp, kidney deficiency, qi deficiency, blood deficiency, etc. Moxibustion to relevant acupoints can dredge meridians, harmonize qi and blood, and effectively improve the symptoms.

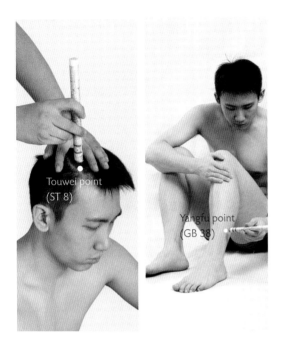

Touwei point
(ST 8)

Yangfu point
(GB 38)

Acupoints of Moxibustion

Moxibustion Method

Mild moxibustion: Moxibustion is applied to the Baihui, Taiyang, Touwei, Shangxing, Yangfu, Taixi, Taichong and Ashi points— Ashi point is the pain point of the disease, which in itself has no fixed location— beginning with the head and then the four limbs. When applying moxibustion to the acupoints on the head, the hair at the acupoint should be parted to both sides so as not to affect the treatment. The practitioner lights one end of a moxa roll and directs the ignited roll head at an acupoint, 3 to 5 centimeters above the surface of the skin. The moxibustion should last 15 to 20 minutes, until the patient feels comfortable and skin near the acupoint turns slightly red. Such treatment should be given once a day; perform two more days after symptoms alleviate.

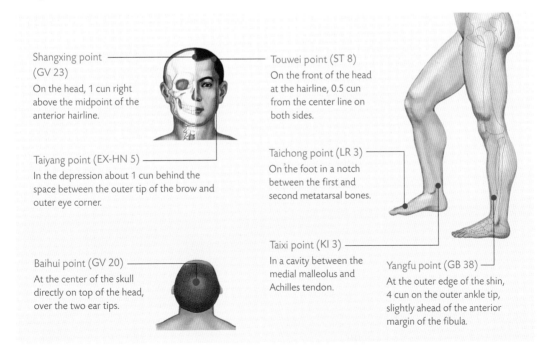

Shangxing point
(GV 23)
On the head, 1 cun right above the midpoint of the anterior hairline.

Touwei point (ST 8)
On the front of the head at the hairline, 0.5 cun from the center line on both sides.

Taiyang point (EX-HN 5)
In the depression about 1 cun behind the space between the outer tip of the brow and outer eye corner.

Taichong point (LR 3)
On the foot in a notch between the first and second metatarsal bones.

Baihui point (GV 20)
At the center of the skull directly on top of the head, over the two ear tips.

Taixi point (KI 3)
In a cavity between the medial malleolus and Achilles tendon.

Yangfu point (GB 38)
At the outer edge of the shin, 4 cun on the outer ankle tip, slightly ahead of the anterior margin of the fibula.

3. Cough

Cough is the main symptom of respiratory diseases. A cough without phlegm or with little phlegm is called a dry cough, and is commonly seen in the acute pharyngitis and the initial stage of bronchitis. An acute cough often appears due to a foreign body in the bronchia, and a long-term chronic cough is most commonly seen in chronic bronchitis inflammation, tuberculosis and other diseases.

Acupoints of Moxibustion

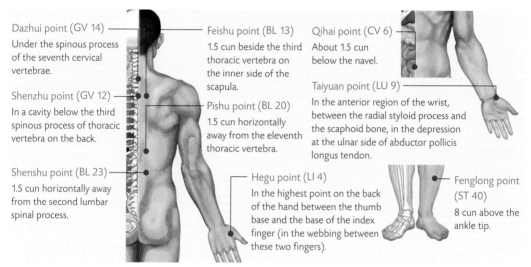

Dazhui point (GV 14)
Under the spinous process of the seventh cervical vertebrae.

Shenzhu point (GV 12)
In a cavity below the third spinous process of thoracic vertebra on the back.

Shenshu point (BL 23)
1.5 cun horizontally away from the second lumbar spinal process.

Feishu point (BL 13)
1.5 cun beside the third thoracic vertebra on the inner side of the scapula.

Pishu point (BL 20)
1.5 cun horizontally away from the eleventh thoracic vertebra.

Hegu point (LI 4)
In the highest point on the back of the hand between the thumb base and the base of the index finger (in the webbing between these two fingers).

Qihai point (CV 6)
About 1.5 cun below the navel.

Taiyuan point (LU 9)
In the anterior region of the wrist, between the radial styloid process and the scaphoid bone, in the depression at the ulnar side of abductor pollicis longus tendon.

Fenglong point (ST 40)
8 cun above the ankle tip.

Moxibustion Methods

Mild moxibustion: Moxibustion is applied to the Feishu, Pishu, Taiyuan, Hegu, and Fenglong points, beginning with upper acupoints and working toward lower acupoints. Let the patient take an appropriate position. The practitioner, standing on one side of the patient, lights one end of a moxa roll and directs the ignited roll head to an acupoint, 3 to 5 centimeters above the surface of the skin, until the patient's local area of skin feels warm but without any burning pain. The patient can apply moxibustion to the accessible points herself as it is more convenient to control the temperature. Moxibustion should last 10 to 15 minutes for each acupoint, until the skin turns slightly red. Such treatment should be given once daily and repeated 5 to 10 times for a course of treatment, with a seven-day interval between two courses. This moxibustion therapy is most suitable for treating phlegm-dampness cough. The symptoms are marked by recurring attacks of cough with noisy and stuffy sounds and lots of phlegm. The cough is caused by phlegm and will be milder or stop if the phlegm is spit out. The phlegm is either sticky or thick, and white or gray in color. A cough becomes

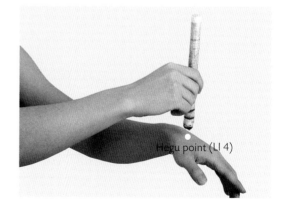

Hegu point (LI 4)

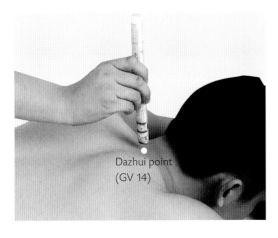

Dazhui point
(GV 14)

serious with increased phlegm mostly in the morning or after a meal. It will be aggravated after the patient eats sweet and oily food, and be accompanied by stuffiness in the chest, fullness in the stomach, vomiting, decreased appetite, fatigue, watery excrement and white tongue-coating.

Mild moxibustion: Moxibustion is applied to the Dazhui, Shenzhu, Feishu, Pishu, Shenshu, Qihai and Fenglong points, beginning with the lower back and then moving on to the chest and abdomen, from upper acupoints to lower acupoints. Let the patient take an appropriate position. The practitioner lights one end of a moxa roll and directs the ignited roll head to an acupoint, 3 to 5 centimeters above the surface of the skin, until the patient's local area of skin feels warm, without the feeling of burning pain. For a patient with diminished sensation, the practitioner can place the index finger and middle finger around the acupoint to feel the skin temperature, so as not to burn the patient's skin. Moxibustion should last 10 to 15 minutes for each acupoint, until the patient's local area of skin turns slightly red. Such treatment should be given once daily or once every other day and repeated 5 to 10 days for a course of treatment with a seven-day interval between two courses. This moxibustion therapy is most suitable for treating qi deficiency cough. The symptoms are emaciation with a sallow complexion, absent-mindedness, cough with clear and light-colored phlegm and reduced appetite.

Ginkgo Nut Chicken Porridge

Ingredients: Rice, chicken breast, ginkgo nuts, appropriate amount of soy sauce, peanut oil, cooking wine, pepper, meat tenderizer and ginger.

Preparation: Mince chicken breast, add soy sauce, peanut oil, cooking wine, pepper, meat tenderizer and ginger, mix and pickle them. Cook a pot of porridge; you can add a few dry shrimps. When the porridge is almost ready, add ginkgo nuts and continue to cook for 10 minutes, then add minced chicken meat until fully cooked. Remove the pot from the heat and add an appropriate amount of salt and sesame oil, and sprinkle with chopped green onions. This porridge is delicious and nutritious and can relieve cough and asthma. Ginkgo nuts are good for moistening the lungs and tonifying qi. They should be cooked and cannot be eaten too much because gingo nut contains ginkgotoxin. Eat no more than eight ginkgo nuts each time.

4. Constipation

Constipation is when the stool stays in the body for a long time, or it is difficult to defecate despite the desire to defecate. A common symptom is significantly reduced frequency of defecation, once every 2 to 3 days or less often, without regularity, and stool that is dry and hard.

Patients suffering from constipation should follow certain dietary principles: Eat more crude fiber foods, choose staple foods that are not too refined, and eat coarse grains. Eat a sufficient amount of vegetables and fruits every day, and drink plenty of water. Develop the habit of defecation at a regular time. Drink a glass of light salt water or honey water every morning, while massaging the abdomen to speed up defecation. Do appropriate physical exercises to regulate organ function and prevent constipation.

Acupoints of Moxibustion

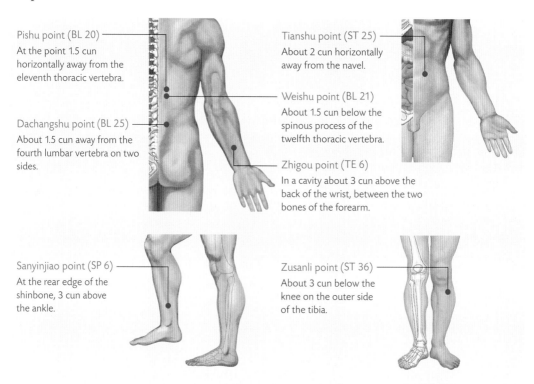

Pishu point (BL 20)
At the point 1.5 cun horizontally away from the eleventh thoracic vertebra.

Dachangshu point (BL 25)
About 1.5 cun away from the fourth lumbar vertebra on two sides.

Tianshu point (ST 25)
About 2 cun horizontally away from the navel.

Weishu point (BL 21)
About 1.5 cun below the spinous process of the twelfth thoracic vertebra.

Zhigou point (TE 6)
In a cavity about 3 cun above the back of the wrist, between the two bones of the forearm.

Sanyinjiao point (SP 6)
At the rear edge of the shinbone, 3 cun above the ankle.

Zusanli point (ST 36)
About 3 cun below the knee on the outer side of the tibia.

Moxibustion Method

Mild moxibustion: Moxibustion is applied to the Pishu, Weishu, Dachangshu, Tianshu, Zhigou, Zusanli and Sanyinjiao points, following the principles of first lower back and then chest and abdomen, working from the upper to lower body. The practitioner, standing on one side of the patient, lights one end of a moxa roll and directs the ignited roll head at an acupoint, 3 to 5 centimeters above the surface of the skin, until the patient's

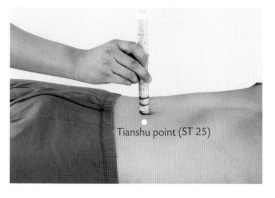

Tianshu point (ST 25)

local area of skin feels warm, without the feeling of burning pain. Moxibustion should last 10 to 15 minutes, until the patient feels comfortable and the acupoint area flushes. Such treatment should be given once daily and repeated 10 times for a course of treatment with a five-day interval between two courses.

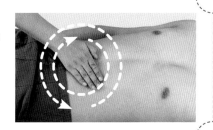

In addition to moxibustion, self-massage is also an effective treatment for constipation. Massage with palm along the navel in clockwise and counterclockwise directions 30 times each, and then gradually spread to the surrounding area and massage the entire abdomen 30 times with the navel as the center. Long-term adherence to this practice will produce good results.

5. Vomit

Vomit is a common clinical symptom, a reflexive action when the stomach contents enter the esophagus and are spit out of the mouth. Its precursory symptom is nausea, and it is also manifested by a discomfort in the upper abdomen, often accompanied by dizziness, salivation, slow pulse, reduced blood pressure, etc. Vomiting is a symptom of gastritis, acute viral hepatitis, acute appendicitis, pyloric obstruction and other diseases.

Diet should be light during treatment, and do not eat raw, cold, greasy, sticky and other indigestible food. Eat more food that can nourish yin and promote the secretion of body fluid, such as millet, flour and various grain products, soybeans, cowpea and other bean products, milk, eggs, lean meat, fish, and other nutritious food that will not produce internal heat in the body, as well as fruits and vegetables.

Acupoints of Moxibustion

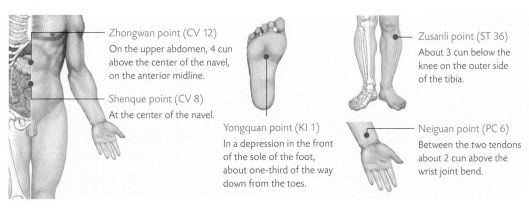

Zhongwan point (CV 12)
On the upper abdomen, 4 cun above the center of the navel, on the anterior midline.

Shenque point (CV 8)
At the center of the navel.

Yongquan point (KI 1)
In a depression in the front of the sole of the foot, about one-third of the way down from the toes.

Zusanli point (ST 36)
About 3 cun below the knee on the outer side of the tibia.

Neiguan point (PC 6)
Between the two tendons about 2 cun above the wrist joint bend.

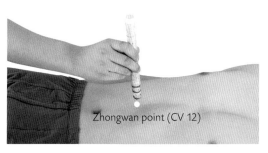

Zhongwan point (CV 12)

Moxibustion Method

Mild moxibustion: Moxibustion is applied to such points as Zhongwan, Shenque, Neiguan, Zusanli and Yongquan, beginning with points on the upper body and then those on the lower body. The patient should take a comfortable posture. The practitioner ignites one end of a moxa roll, and points the ignited end at a point, 3 to 5 centimeters above the skin's surface, until the patient's local skin feels warm, without the feeling of burning pain. It's advisable for the patient to perform moxibustion to accessible points by himself to more easily control the temperature. Moxibustion lasts 15 to 20 minutes for each point, until the patient's local skin turns red. Moxibustion should be performed once or twice a day and continue one more day after the symptoms alleviate.

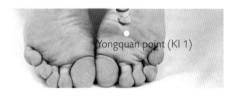
Yongquan point (KI 1)

1. Wild Chrysanthemum Tea

Ingredients: 1.1 ounces of wild chrysanthemums, appropriate amount of sugar.

Preparation: Boil the wild chrysanthemums, leave the juice after removing the slag, and add an appropriate amount of sugar. Drink this tea several times a day for three days.

2. Fried Lean Meat with Bitter Gourd

Ingredients: Bitter gourd, lean meat.

Preparation: Fry appropriate amount of bitter gourd and lean meat in a pan. Eat it as a dish, once a day.

3. Cold Dish

Ingredients: One cucumber, one carrot, two Chinese cabbage leaves.

Preparation: Cut the cucumber, carrot and Chinese cabbage leaves into slices, and mix them into a cold dish. Eat this dish once a day.

6. Hiccups

Hiccups are a phenomenon in which qi adversely flows from the stomach, and frequently leads to quick and short sounds in the throat. It is a physiologically common phenomenon caused by the contradiction of diaphragmatic tendons. Hiccups resulting from the overeating and overdrinking or hot or cold irritation can be automatically relieved, but hiccups caused by diseases should be treated actively.

Moxibustion Methods

Sparrow-pecking moxibustion:
Moxibustion is applied to such points as Geshu, Tiantu, Danzhong, Zhongwan, Liangmen, Neiguan and Zusanli, moving from the points on the waist and back and

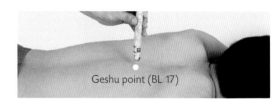
Geshu point (BL 17)

to those on the chest and abdomen. Work from the upper to lower body. Ignite one end of a moxa roll and point the ignited end at a point, keeping it 2 to 3 centimeters from the skin's surface, and move it up and down like a bird pecking at food. Each point is given the therapy for 10 to 20 minutes, once or twice a day and one more day after the symptoms alleviate. This method is effective on hiccups caused by cold in the stomach. The symptoms are slow and forceful hiccups along with discomfort in the stomach. These symptoms will be reduced when the stomach is warmed up and will be aggravated when the stomach gets cold. The patient does not feel thirsty and has a white tongue surface and slow pulse.

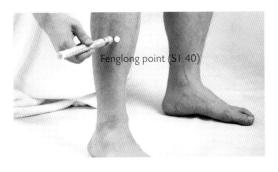
Fenglong point (ST 40)

Mild moxibustion: Moxibustion is applied to such points as Geshu, Qimen, Tianshu, Neiguan, Fenglong and Taichong, beginning with points on the waist and back and then moving to those on the chest and abdomen, working from the upper to lower body. The patient should take an appropriate posture. Ignite a moxa roll at one end and point the ignited end at a point, staying 3 to 5 centimeters above the skin's surface, until the local skin feels warm but no burning pain. Moxibustion of the Fenglong and Taichong points can be performed by the patients themselves so as to control the temperature. Moxibustion lasts 15 to 20 minutes for each point, until the local skin turns slightly red. The therapy should be applied once or twice a day and continue one more day after the symptoms alleviate. This method is effective on hiccups caused by stagnation of qi and blockage of sputa. The symptoms are continuous hiccups with stuffiness in the chest, weak appetite, nausea, rumbling intestines, difficulty breathing, poor eyesight, dizziness, increased phlegm and a thin and sticky tongue coating.

Acupoints of Moxibustion

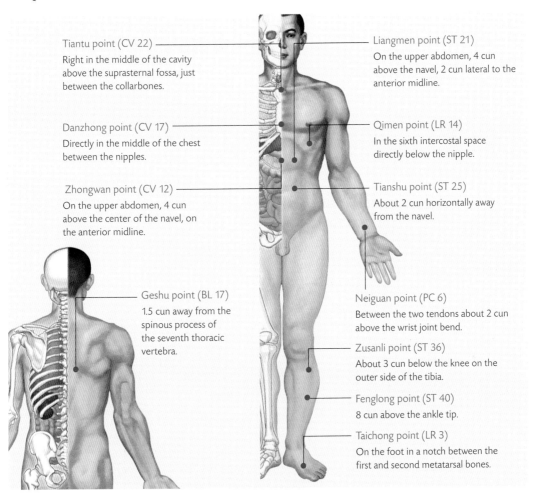

Tiantu point (CV 22)
Right in the middle of the cavity above the suprasternal fossa, just between the collarbones.

Danzhong point (CV 17)
Directly in the middle of the chest between the nipples.

Zhongwan point (CV 12)
On the upper abdomen, 4 cun above the center of the navel, on the anterior midline.

Geshu point (BL 17)
1.5 cun away from the spinous process of the seventh thoracic vertebra.

Liangmen point (ST 21)
On the upper abdomen, 4 cun above the navel, 2 cun lateral to the anterior midline.

Qimen point (LR 14)
In the sixth intercostal space directly below the nipple.

Tianshu point (ST 25)
About 2 cun horizontally away from the navel.

Neiguan point (PC 6)
Between the two tendons about 2 cun above the wrist joint bend.

Zusanli point (ST 36)
About 3 cun below the knee on the outer side of the tibia.

Fenglong point (ST 40)
8 cun above the ankle tip.

Taichong point (LR 3)
On the foot in a notch between the first and second metatarsal bones.

7. Abdominal Pain

Abdominal pain is a pathological change of internal and external abdominal organs with various causes. Abdominal pain is divided into acute and chronic cases. The reasons for this condition are extremely complex, including inflammation, tumors, bleeding, obstruction, perforation, trauma and dysfunction.

Patients with abdominal pain should pay attention to adjusting their diets, and should not eat and drink too much, should not eat raw, cold or irritating food, but should eat more easily digestible fruits and vegetables. They should not rush to exercise after a meal, and should pay attention to warming the abdomen because abdominal cold can easily lead to abdominal pain. Patients need to avoid mental stress or depression, and to maintain peace of mind, which can help relieve symptoms and alleviate abdominal pain. They should have appropriate exercise to enhance organs function and improve disease resistance.

Acupoints of Moxibustion

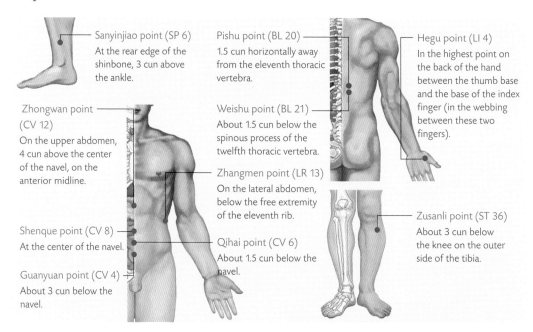

Sanyinjiao point (SP 6)
At the rear edge of the shinbone, 3 cun above the ankle.

Zhongwan point (CV 12)
On the upper abdomen, 4 cun above the center of the navel, on the anterior midline.

Shenque point (CV 8)
At the center of the navel.

Guanyuan point (CV 4)
About 3 cun below the navel.

Pishu point (BL 20)
1.5 cun horizontally away from the eleventh thoracic vertebra.

Weishu point (BL 21)
About 1.5 cun below the spinous process of the twelfth thoracic vertebra.

Zhangmen point (LR 13)
On the lateral abdomen, below the free extremity of the eleventh rib.

Qihai point (CV 6)
About 1.5 cun below the navel.

Hegu point (LI 4)
In the highest point on the back of the hand between the thumb base and the base of the index finger (in the webbing between these two fingers).

Zusanli point (ST 36)
About 3 cun below the knee on the outer side of the tibia.

Moxibustion Method

Mild moxibustion: Moxibustion is applied to the Pishu, Weishu, Zhongwan, Zhangmen, Shenque, Qihai, Guanyuan, Zusanli, Sanyinjiao and Hegu points, beginning with the points on the waist and back and then moving to those on the chest and abdomen, working from the upper to lower body. The patient should take a comfortable posture. The practitioner ignites one end of a moxa roll and points the ignited end at a point,

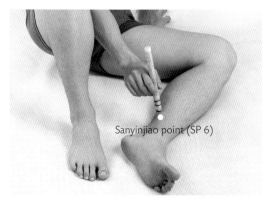

Sanyinjiao point (SP 6)

3 to 5 centimeters above the skin's surface, until the patient's local skin feels warm, without the feeling of burning pain. The patient can apply moxibustion to the accessible points by herself for best temperature control. Apply moxibustion 10 to 15 minutes for each point, until the patient feels comfortable and their local skin turns slightly red. Such treatment should be performed once a day and continue 1 to 2 days more after the symptoms alleviate.

8. Diarrhea

Diarrhea is a manifestation of tenuous stools and an increase in the frequency of defecation. It is divided into acute and chronic diarrhea. Acute diarrhea has a sudden onset and lasts for 2 to 3 weeks, while chronic diarrhea lasts for more than 2 months or recurs frequently in an intermittent period of 2 to 4 weeks.

According to traditional Chinese medicine, acute diarrhea is usually caused by exogenous pathogens or eating and drinking, and chronic diarrhea is caused by deficiency of the spleen and stomach. Moxibustion at relevant points can expel pathogenic cold, regulate spleen and stomach, and relieve symptoms.

When a person loses a lot of water during diarrhea, it's important to increase the intake of liquid or semi-liquid in the diet, including milk, lotus root starch, vegetable juice, fruit juice, egg soup, soft noodles and gruel. These are easy to digest and absorb and contain the electrolytes the human body needs. Patients should also pay attention to rest and avoid overwork, so as not to aggravate the conditions. They should not use drugs such as antibiotics indiscriminately, and those in severe conditions should seek medical treatment.

Acupoints of Moxibustion

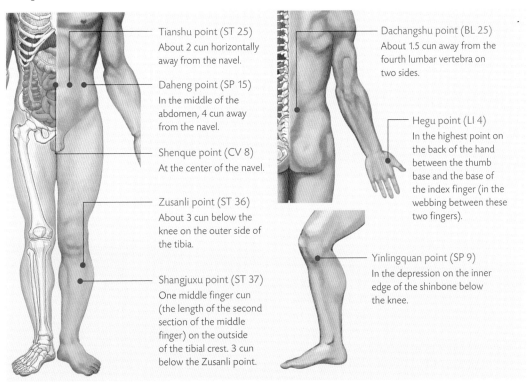

Tianshu point (ST 25)
About 2 cun horizontally away from the navel.

Daheng point (SP 15)
In the middle of the abdomen, 4 cun away from the navel.

Shenque point (CV 8)
At the center of the navel.

Zusanli point (ST 36)
About 3 cun below the knee on the outer side of the tibia.

Shangjuxu point (ST 37)
One middle finger cun (the length of the second section of the middle finger) on the outside of the tibial crest. 3 cun below the Zusanli point.

Dachangshu point (BL 25)
About 1.5 cun away from the fourth lumbar vertebra on two sides.

Hegu point (LI 4)
In the highest point on the back of the hand between the thumb base and the base of the index finger (in the webbing between these two fingers).

Yinlingquan point (SP 9)
In the depression on the inner edge of the shinbone below the knee.

Moxibustion Method

Mild moxibustion: Moxibustion is applied to the Dachangshu, Shenque, Tianshu, Daheng, Zusanli, Shangjuxu, Yinlingquan and Hegu points, beginning with points on the waist and back and then moving to those on the chest and abdomen, working from the upper to lower body. The patient should take an appropriate posture. The practitioner ignites a moxa roll at one end and points it accurately at a point, with the ignited end 3 to 5 centimeters from the skin's surface, until the patient feels warmth but no pain. For a patient with reduced sensitivity, the practitioner can place index and middle fingers near the point to feel the temperature, so as not to burn the patient's skin. Moxibustion lasts 15 to 30 minutes for each point, until the local skin of the patient turns slightly red. Such treatment should be performed once or twice a day and continue 1 to 2 more days after symptoms alleviate.

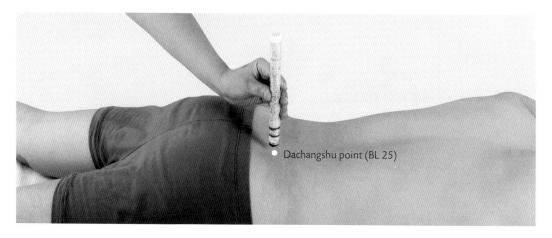

Dachangshu point (BL 25)

9. Heartburn

Heartburn is caused by the reflux of stomach contents into the esophagus. The symptoms are burning pain in the upper abdomen or lower chest, accompanied by sour regurgitation. It is a common disease of the digestive system. The most frequent reason for heartburn is eating too fast or too much.

According to traditional Chinese medicine, heartburn can be easily caused by excessive drinking or eating too much spicy or high-fat food. Moxibustion at relevant points can improve the body's immunity and enhance disease resistance.

Moxibustion Method

Mild moxibustion: Moxibustion is applied to such points as Pishu, Weishu, Zhongwan, Neiguan, Zusanli and Gongsun, beginning with the points on the waist and back and then moving to those on the chest and abdomen, and working from the upper to lower body. The patient should take an appropriate posture. The practitioner

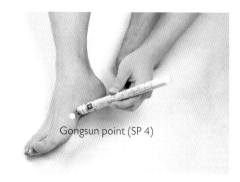

Gongsun point (SP 4)

ignites a moxa roll at one end and points it accurately at a point, with the ignited end 3 to 5 centimeters above the skin's surface, until the patient feels targeted warmth but no burning pain. It's ideal for the patient is to apply moxibustion to accessible points himself for the best temperature control. Moxibustion lasts 15 to 20 minutes for each point, until the local skin turns slightly red. Such treatment should be given once a day, and 10 times for a course of treatment with an interval of one or two days between two courses.

Acupoints of Moxibustion

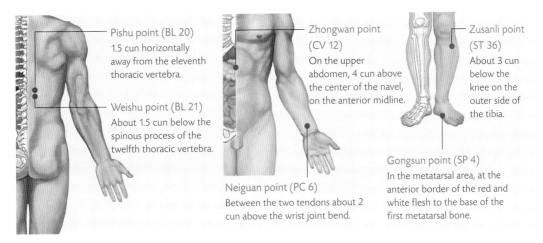

Pishu point (BL 20)
1.5 cun horizontally away from the eleventh thoracic vertebra.

Weishu point (BL 21)
About 1.5 cun below the spinous process of the twelfth thoracic vertebra.

Zhongwan point (CV 12)
On the upper abdomen, 4 cun above the center of the navel, on the anterior midline.

Neiguan point (PC 6)
Between the two tendons about 2 cun above the wrist joint bend.

Zusanli point (ST 36)
About 3 cun below the knee on the outer side of the tibia.

Gongsun point (SP 4)
In the metatarsal area, at the anterior border of the red and white flesh to the base of the first metatarsal bone.

10. Bacterial Dysentery

Bacterial dysentery, abbreviated as dysentery, is an infectious intestinal disease caused by shigella dysenteriae. Its clinical manifestations are cold, fever, abdominal pain, diarrhea, tenesmus, and stools containing pus and blood. In the case of toxic dysentery, patients will have such symptoms as high fever, convulsions and coma. Moxibustion at the relevant points can eliminate dampness and heat and replenish the spleen and stomach.

Acupoints of Moxibustion

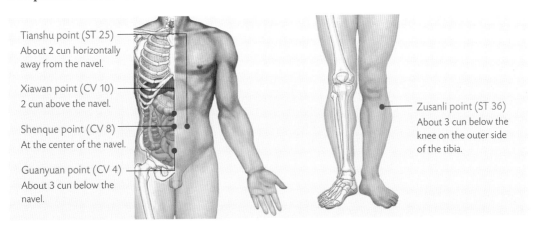

Tianshu point (ST 25)
About 2 cun horizontally away from the navel.

Xiawan point (CV 10)
2 cun above the navel.

Shenque point (CV 8)
At the center of the navel.

Guanyuan point (CV 4)
About 3 cun below the navel.

Zusanli point (ST 36)
About 3 cun below the knee on the outer side of the tibia.

Moxibustion Method

Mild moxibustion: Moxibustion is applied to the Xiawan, Shenque, Tianshu, Guanyuan and Zusanli points, moving from points on the upper body to those on the lower body. The patient should take an appropriate posture. The practitioner, standing on one side of the patient, ignites a moxa roll at one end and points it accurately at a point, with the ignited end 3 to 5 centimeters above the skin's surface, until the local skin of the patient feels warm, without the feeling of burning pain. Apply moxibustion 5 minutes per point, until local skin turns slightly red. Such treatment should be given once a day and repeated five times for a course of treatment with a one-day interval between two courses.

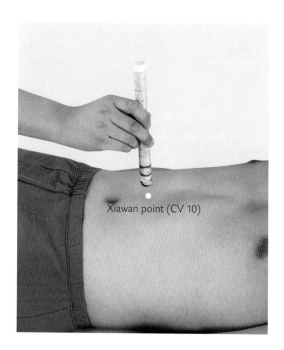

Xiawan point (CV 10)

11. Gastroptosis

Gastroptosis refers to a condition in which the lower border of the stomach reaches the pelvic cavity while standing, and the lowest point of the lesser curvature of the stomach is below the line connecting the crista iliaca. Mild cases of gastroptosis are usually asymptomatic, but severe ones may cause such symptoms as abdominal distention, abdominal pain, nausea, vomiting and constipation.

Acupoints of Moxibustion

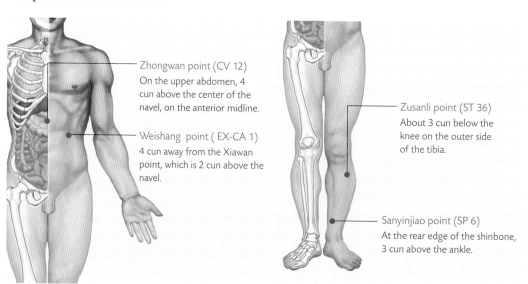

Zhongwan point (CV 12)
On the upper abdomen, 4 cun above the center of the navel, on the anterior midline.

Weishang point (EX-CA 1)
4 cun away from the Xiawan point, which is 2 cun above the navel.

Zusanli point (ST 36)
About 3 cun below the knee on the outer side of the tibia.

Sanyinjiao point (SP 6)
At the rear edge of the shinbone, 3 cun above the ankle.

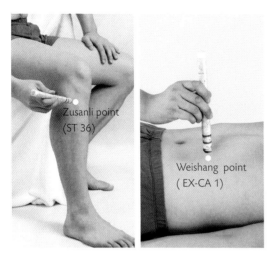

Zusanli point
(ST 36)

Weishang point
(EX-CA 1)

Moxibustion Method

Mild moxibustion: Moxibustion is applied to the Zusanli, Sanyinjiao, Zhongwan and Weishang points, beginning with points on the upper body and then moving to those on the lower body. The patient should take an appropriate posture. The practitioner ignites one end of a moxa roll and points the ignited end at a point, 3 to 5 centimeters above the skin's surface, until the skin feels warm but not burning. The patient should perform moxibustion on Zusanli and Sanyinjiao points herself for the best temperature control. Moxibustion lasts 15 to 20 minutes for each point, until the skin turns slightly red. Such treatment should be given once or twice a day, 10 times as a course of treatment, with an interval of 3 to 5 days between two courses.

12. Nosebleed

Nosebleed refers to blood flowing from the nostrils after the vessels have been damaged due to the fragility of blood capillary of the nasal mucosa. Nosebleeds are one-sided in most cases, but sometimes two-sided. They recur intermittently, and persistently. The amount of bleeding ranges from nasal mucus with blood in mild cases to hemorrhagic shock in severe cases. Repeated bleeding can lead to anemia. In most cases, bleeding can cease spontaneously.

Acupoints of Moxibustion

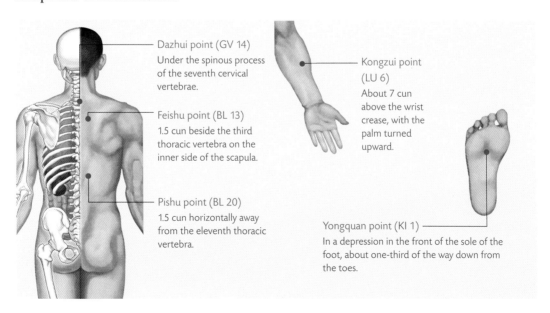

Dazhui point (GV 14)
Under the spinous process of the seventh cervical vertebrae.

Feishu point (BL 13)
1.5 cun beside the third thoracic vertebra on the inner side of the scapula.

Pishu point (BL 20)
1.5 cun horizontally away from the eleventh thoracic vertebra.

Kongzui point (LU 6)
About 7 cun above the wrist crease, with the palm turned upward.

Yongquan point (KI 1)
In a depression in the front of the sole of the foot, about one-third of the way down from the toes.

Moxibustion Method

Mild moxibustion: Moxibustion is applied to the Dazhui, Feishu, Pishu, Yongquan and Kongzui points, moving from the upper to lower body. The patient should take an appropriate posture. The practitioner ignites a moxa roll at one end and points the ignited end accurately at a point, 3 to 5 centimeters above the skin's surface, until the targeted skin of the patient feels warm but not burning. Moxibustion lasts 15 to 20 minutes per point, until the patient's skin turns slightly red. Such treatment is given once or twice a day and continues 1 to 3 more days after symptoms alleviate. During moxibustion, the practitioner should be sure to keep falling ash from burning the skin.

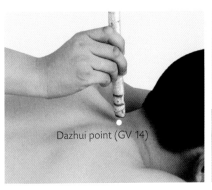

Dazhui point (GV 14)

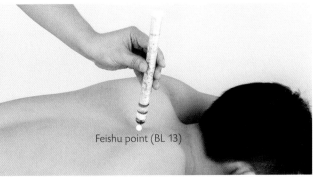

Feishu point (BL 13)

13. Hypotension

Hypotension is low blood pressure. Mild hypotension can cause dizziness, headache, anorexia, fatigue, a pallid complexion, indigestion or motion sickness, while a more severe version can lead to orthostatic dizziness, cold limbs, palpitations, dyspnea and other symptoms. Long-term hypotension can greatly reduce the body functions and induce other diseases.

Hypotensive patients should pay attention to diet combination, and eat more longan, lotus seeds, Chinese dates, mulberries, etc., to enhance the brain function and improve health. They should choose food rich in protein, iron, copper, and with high cholesterol, such as liver, eggs and fish. Do not eat cold or qi-consuming food, such as radishes, celery and cold drinks. Hypotensive patients can benefit from physical exercise to improve their fitness.

Moxibustion Method

Mild moxibustion: Moxibustion is applied to the Zusanli and Sanyinjiao points. Moxibustion of these two points can be performed by the patient himself to control the temperature. Take a comfortable posture. Ignite a moxa roll at one end and point the ignited end at a point, 3 to 5 centimeters

Acupoints of Moxibustion

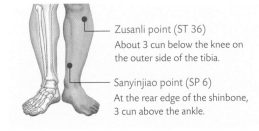

Zusanli point (ST 36)
About 3 cun below the knee on the outer side of the tibia.

Sanyinjiao point (SP 6)
At the rear edge of the shinbone, 3 cun above the ankle.

above the skin's surface, until local skin feels warm but not burning pain. Moxibustion lasts 15 to 20 minutes per point until the local skin turns slightly red. The treatment is given once or twice a day and continues 3 to 5 more days after symptoms alleviate.

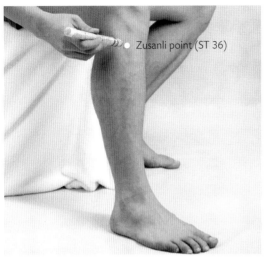

Zusanli point (ST 36)

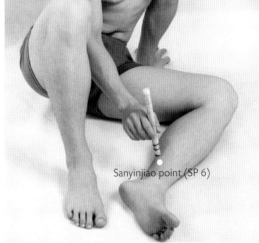

Sanyinjiao point (SP 6)

14. Dizziness

Dizziness is a disease mainly characterized by a whirling sensation in the head and blurred eyes. The condition is generally considered a subjective sensation caused by a person's spatial orientation disorder, and an illusion in the judgment of her surroundings and position. Dizziness that includes a whirling sensation, a floating sensation, and a lifting and dropping sensation is more serious than general dizziness. There are many causes for dizziness; when the condition occurs, visit a doctor for a physical exam.

Acupoints of Moxibustion

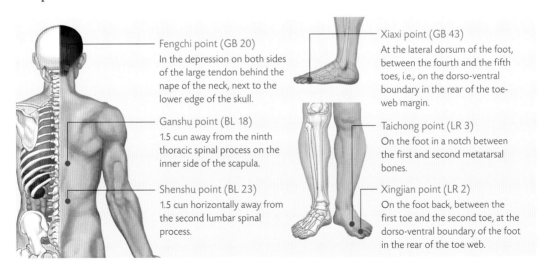

Fengchi point (GB 20)
In the depression on both sides of the large tendon behind the nape of the neck, next to the lower edge of the skull.

Ganshu point (BL 18)
1.5 cun away from the ninth thoracic spinal process on the inner side of the scapula.

Shenshu point (BL 23)
1.5 cun horizontally away from the second lumbar spinal process.

Xiaxi point (GB 43)
At the lateral dorsum of the foot, between the fourth and the fifth toes, i.e., on the dorso-ventral boundary in the rear of the toe-web margin.

Taichong point (LR 3)
On the foot in a notch between the first and second metatarsal bones.

Xingjian point (LR 2)
On the foot back, between the first toe and the second toe, at the dorso-ventral boundary of the foot in the rear of the toe web.

Moxibustion Method

Mild moxibustion: Moxibustion is applied to the Fengchi, Ganshu, Shenshu, Xiaxi, Xingjian and Taichong points, moving from the upper to lower body. The patient should take an appropriate posture. The practitioner ignites one end of a moxa roll and points the ignited end at a point, 3 to 5 centimeters above the skin's surface, until the patient feels warm, without the feeling of burning pain. Moxibustion lasts 15 to 30 minutes for each point, until the local skin turns slightly red. When performing moxibustion on the Fengchi point, you can place a piece of ginger on the point to prevent ash from falling onto the hair. Such treatment should be given once a day or once every other day for a 10-day course of treatment, with an interval of 3 to 5 days between two courses.

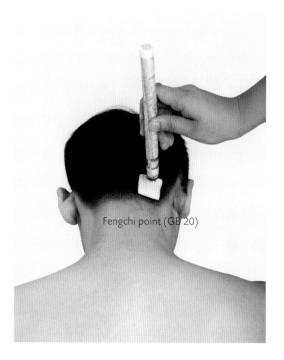

Fengchi point (GB 20)

15. Toothache

Toothache is a common symptom among oral diseases with a variety of causes such as dental caries, pulpitis, periapical inflammation and dentine hypersensitivity. Toothaches can be induced or aggravated by a variety of stimuli such as cold, heat, and acidic or sweet food.

Patients should pay attention to oral hygiene and develop a good habit of toothbrushing in the morning and in the evening and rinsing the mouth after meals. They should eat more food that serves to clear away the stomach and liver fire, such as pumpkin, watermelon, water chestnut, celery and radish. They should not drink alcohol and should not eat heat-inducing or hard food, and should eat less sour, frozen or overheated food. They should reduce or control the amount of sugar in the food and seek timely medical treatment if there is a dental disease.

Acupoints of Moxibustion

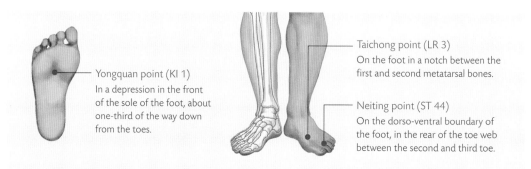

Yongquan point (KI 1)
In a depression in the front of the sole of the foot, about one-third of the way down from the toes.

Taichong point (LR 3)
On the foot in a notch between the first and second metatarsal bones.

Neiting point (ST 44)
On the dorso-ventral boundary of the foot, in the rear of the toe web between the second and third toe.

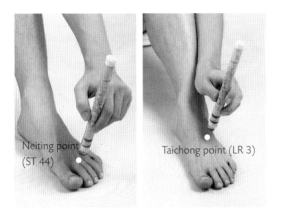

Neiting point (ST 44)

Taichong point (LR 3)

Moxibustion Method

Sparrow-pecking moxibustion:
Moxibustion is applied to such points as Yongquan, Neiting and Taichong. While the patient takes an appropriate posture, the practitioner ignites one end of a moxa roll and points the ignited end accurately at a point, about 3 centimeters above the skin's surface, and moves it up and down like a bird pecking at food. Moxibustion lasts 5 minutes per point. This is performed once or twice a day, and lasts one or two more days after symptoms alleviate. This method is characterized by the sudden drop and rise in temperature and has quite a strong effect of arousing the functions of points and meridians.

16. Oral Ulcers

Oral ulcer is a kind of superficial ulcer on the oral mucosa characterized by periodic recurrence. Ulcers can develop in any part of the oral mucosa and can recover spontaneously. The causes of oral ulcers include local trauma, mental stress, food, drugs and change in hormone levels, as well as deficiency of vitamins or microelements. According to the Western medicine, oral ulcers are mostly caused by viruses.

Patients with oral ulcers should pay attention to daily oral hygiene, frequently rinsing the mouth with light salt water and often moistening the mouth to avoid dry mouth. They should also drink plenty of water and eat zinc-containing foods like lean meat, eggs, peanuts and walnuts to promote wound healing. Eating more foods rich in vitamins B1, B2 and C can help ulcers heal. Therefore, patients should eat more fresh vegetables and fruits such as tomato, eggplant, carrot, white radish, cabbage and spinach. They should avoid spicy food and foods that can cause excessive internal heat such as peppers and mutton. Avoid smoking, alcohol, coffee and irritating drinks.

Acupoints of Moxibustion

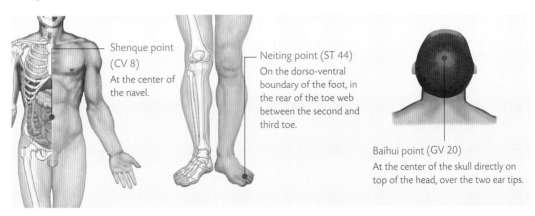

Shenque point (CV 8)
At the center of the navel.

Neiting point (ST 44)
On the dorso-ventral boundary of the foot, in the rear of the toe web between the second and third toe.

Baihui point (GV 20)
At the center of the skull directly on top of the head, over the two ear tips.

Moxibustion Method

Sparrow-pecking moxibustion:
Moxibustion is applied to the Baihui, Shenque and Neiting points, moving from the upper to lower body. The patient should take a comfortable posture. The practitioner ignites a moxa roll and points the ignited end at a point, about 3 centimeters above the skin's surface. The practitioner moves the moxa roll up and down, like a sparrow pecking at food. Moxibustion lasts 5 minutes per point, until local skin turns slightly red. It is performed once every day, for three times as a course of treatment, with an interval of 1 to 2 days between two courses. This method

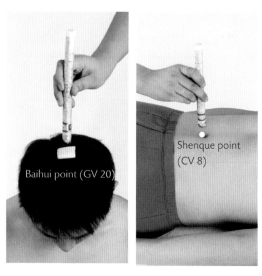

Baihui point (GV 20)

Shenque point (CV 8)

is characterized by the sudden drop and rise in temperature and has a quite strong effect of arousing the functions of points and meridians. Place a slice of ginger over the Baihui point when moxibustion is applied to to prevent ash from falling onto the hair.

1. Chinese Cabbage Root Tea with Garlic Sprouts and Chinese Dates
Ingredients: 2.1 ounces of Chinese cabbage roots, 0.5 ounce of garlic sprouts, and ten Chinese dates.
    Preparation: Decoct Chinese cabbage roots, garlic sprouts, and Chinese dates with water, and drink once or twice a day. This is conducive to the cure of oral ulcers.

2. Fungus Hawthorn Tea
Ingredients: 0.4 ounce each of white fungus, black fungus and hawthorn fruits.
    Preparation: Decoct white fungus, black fungus and hawthorn fruits with water. Drink the tea and eat the fungus once or twice a day. This is conducive to the cure of oral ulcers.

3. Apple Therapy
Ingredients: An apple, a moderate amount of wine.
    Preparation: Cut the apple (or pear) into pieces and place them to a container, and then add enough cold water to submerge the apple or pear, and heat to boiling. After the soup becomes slightly cool, keep the apple or pear slices in the mouth together with wine for a while before eating them. The symptoms can be cured by using this treatment several days in a row.

17. Chronic Rhinitis

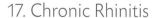

Chronic rhinitis is a chronic inflammation of the nasal mucosa and submucosa, manifested as chronic congestion and swelling of the nasal mucosa. The main symptoms are nasal congestion, runny nose and olfactory disturbance.

    Patients with chronic rhinitis should pay attention to diet regulation and eat less spicy and fried foods such as pepper, ginger and fritters. At the same time, they should also eat less seafood and more vitamin-rich vegetables and fruits such as apples, cabbage, spinach and carrots. Patients should avoid catching a cold since it can cause or aggravate rhinitis, and they should pay attention to the balance of work and rest, avoiding overworking themselves or staying up late. They should actively take physical exercise to enhance their disease resistance.

Acupoints of Moxibustion

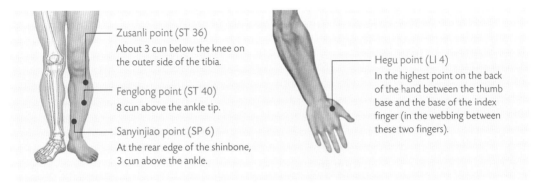

Zusanli point (ST 36)
About 3 cun below the knee on the outer side of the tibia.

Fenglong point (ST 40)
8 cun above the ankle tip.

Sanyinjiao point (SP 6)
At the rear edge of the shinbone, 3 cun above the ankle.

Hegu point (LI 4)
In the highest point on the back of the hand between the thumb base and the base of the index finger (in the webbing between these two fingers).

Moxibustion Method

Swirling moxibustion: Moxibustion is applied to the Zusanli, Sanyinjiao, Fenglong and Hegu points, moving from the upper to the lower body. Moxibustion of these points can be performed by patients themselves or with the help of their family members. Take an appropriate posture. Ignite one end of a moxa roll and point the ignited end at a point, about 3 centimeters above the skin's surface. Then move the ignited end over the point left and right, or circularly, with the range of movement not too large and kept within about 3 centimeters, until it brings mild warmth without the feeling of burning pain on the skin. The moxibustion lasts 10 to 15 minutes per point. This is performed once every day, for 10 times as a course of treatment, with an interval of 3 to 5 days between two courses.

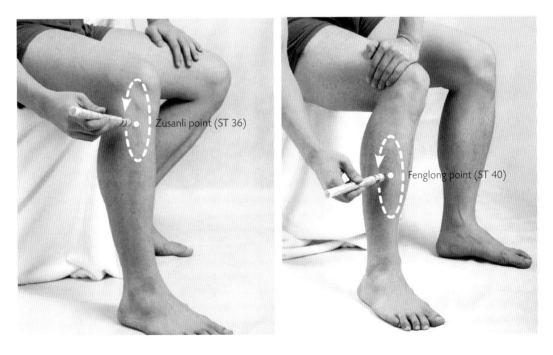

Zusanli point (ST 36)

Fenglong point (ST 40)

18. Sinusitis

Sinusitis is a nonspecific inflammation of the paranasal sinus mucosa, which is a common nasal disease. There are two types of sinusitis: acute and chronic. Acute suppurative sinusitis is mostly secondary to acute rhinitis, mainly characterized by nasal congestion, purulent nasal discharge and headache. Chronic suppurative sinusitis is often secondary to acute suppurative sinusitis and mainly characterized by purulent nasal discharge and can be accompanied by varying levels of nasal congestion, headache and olfactory disturbance.

Acupoints of Moxibustion

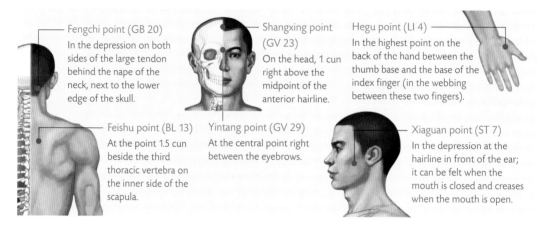

Fengchi point (GB 20)
In the depression on both sides of the large tendon behind the nape of the neck, next to the lower edge of the skull.

Shangxing point (GV 23)
On the head, 1 cun right above the midpoint of the anterior hairline.

Hegu point (LI 4)
In the highest point on the back of the hand between the thumb base and the base of the index finger (in the webbing between these two fingers).

Feishu point (BL 13)
At the point 1.5 cun beside the third thoracic vertebra on the inner side of the scapula.

Yintang point (GV 29)
At the central point right between the eyebrows.

Xiaguan point (ST 7)
In the depression at the hairline in front of the ear; it can be felt when the mouth is closed and creases when the mouth is open.

Moxibustion Method

Swirling moxibustion: Moxibustion is applied to such points as Shangxing, Yintang, Feishu, Fengchi, Xiaguan and Hegu, beginning with points on the head and then those on the limbs, moving from the upper to lower body. The patient should take a comfortable posture. The practitioner ignites a moxa roll at one end and points the ignited end at a point, about 3 centimeters from the skin's surface, and then moves the roll left and right, or circularly, until the skin feels warm but without burning pain. The movement should not be too fast, to avoid possible burn injury or ignition of fabrics caused by falling ash. The movement range should be maintained at about 3 centimeters. The moxibustion lasts 10 to 15 minutes per point. This is performed once every day, 10 times for a course of treatment, with an interval of 3 to 5 days between two courses.

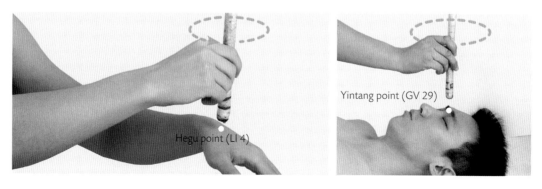

Hegu point (LI 4)

Yintang point (GV 29)

19. Chronic Pharyngitis

Chronic pharyngitis refers to diffuse pharyngeal lesions caused by chronic infections. It is more common in adults and is often accompanied by other respiratory diseases. The most common symptoms are foreign body sensation, slight itching, and dryness with a burning sensation in the pharynx. It is often accompanied by thick viscous secretions attached to the posterior pharyngeal wall that are difficult to clear up, with patient making a "squeak" sound, especially at night. Secretions can cause an irritating cough or even nausea and vomiting.

Patients with pharyngitis should use dietary conditioning by eating light and easily digestible food, as well as eating more cool and refreshing food that can reduce internal heat, and fresh, tender and juicy food. Tobacco, wine, ginger, pepper, mustard, garlic and all spicy things should be avoided. Maintaining proper indoor temperature and humidity is an effective measure to prevent chronic pharyngitis. Develop good oral hygiene habits, gargle after meals and brush your teeth in the morning and evening to keep the mouth clean. At the same time, prevention and treatment of oral and nasal diseases as well as elimination of inflammatory lesions is also important to the prevention and treatment of pharyngitis.

Acupoints of Moxibustion

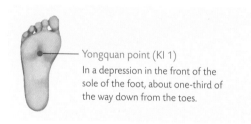

Yongquan point (KI 1)
In a depression in the front of the sole of the foot, about one-third of the way down from the toes.

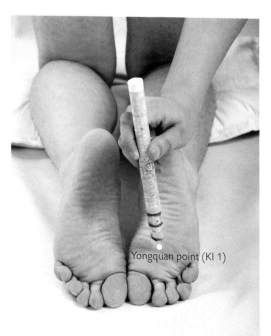

Yongquan point (KI 1)

Moxibustion Method

Mild moxibustion: Treatment is applied to the Yongquan point. The patient should take a prone posture, with the soles of the feet exposed. The practitioner ignites a moxa roll at one end and points the ignited end at a point, 3 to 5 centimeters from the skin's surface, until the patient's skin feels warmth, without a feeling of burning pain. For a patient with decreased sensitivity, the practitioner can place the index finger and middle finger around the point to feel the skin temperature, so as not to burn the patient. Apply moxibustion to the Yongquan point for 15 to 30 minutes, until local skin turns slightly red. This is performed once or twice a day, 10 times for a course of treatment, with an interval of 3 to 5 days between two courses.

The Yongquan point is a point located on the Shaoyin Kidney Meridian of Feet (KI), and is at the lowest part of the body. Moxibustion over this point can cure diseases by leading internal fire from the top of the meridians downward. Moxibustion has an effect of warming yang, thus moxibustion on the Yongquan point has the dual effect of nourishing the kidneys to strengthen yang and inducing the fire back to its origin.

20. Acute Tonsillitis

Acute tonsillitis is a nonspecific acute inflammation of the palatine tonsils, often accompanied by a certain degree of acute inflammation of the pharyngeal mucosa and pharyngeal lymphoid tissues. It often occurs in children and adolescents. It attacks suddenly, and the main symptoms are aversion to cold and a high fever (body temperature may reach 102 to 104°F, and especially small children might suffer from convulsions, vomiting or lethargic sleep due to high fever), lack of appetite, constipation, aching and tiredness in the body.

Acupoints of Moxibustion

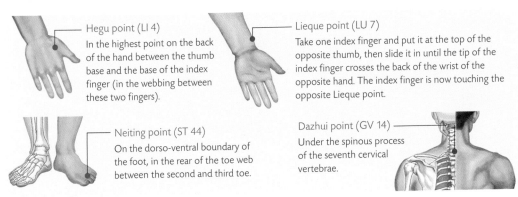

Hegu point (LI 4)
In the highest point on the back of the hand between the thumb base and the base of the index finger (in the webbing between these two fingers).

Lieque point (LU 7)
Take one index finger and put it at the top of the opposite thumb, then slide it in until the tip of the index finger crosses the back of the wrist of the opposite hand. The index finger is now touching the opposite Lieque point.

Neiting point (ST 44)
On the dorso-ventral boundary of the foot, in the rear of the toe web between the second and third toe.

Dazhui point (GV 14)
Under the spinous process of the seventh cervical vertebrae.

Moxibustion Method

Swirling moxibustion: Moxibustion is applied to the Hegu, Lieque, Neiting and Dazhui points, moving from the upper to lower body. The practitioner ignites a moxa roll and points the ignited end at a point, about 3 centimeters above the skin. Then the practitioner holds the roll and moves it left and right or circularly, within a movement range of about 3 centimeters. Moxibustion lasts 15 to 20 minutes, until the skin becomes red. The moxibustion should be given once a day for a five-day course of treatment, with a three-day interval between two courses.

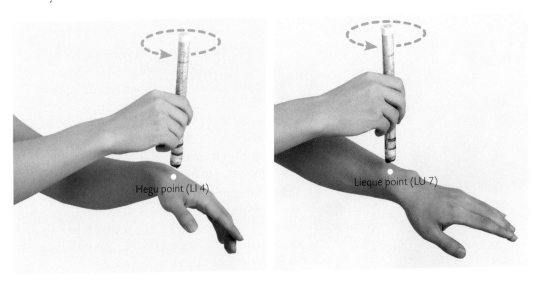

Hegu point (LI 4)

Lieque point (LU 7)

21. Pseudomyopia

Pseudomyopia is the spasm of the ciliary muscle, increased lens thickness and blurred vision caused by excessive use of the eyes. If not relieved in a timely fashion, the intense pressure on eyeballs from the extraocular muscles can eventually cause true myopia as the axial length increases.

Pseudomyopia should be treated actively so it doesn't develop into true myopia. Patients should pay attention to improving the learning environment and maintaining a correct posture while reading and writing. Pay attention to light and ensure adequate lighting in the room. Keep an appropriate balance between work and rest, get rid of bad study habits, and do not read while lying down or walking. Pay attention to strengthening physical exercise. Eat more food containing chromium and zinc, such as soybeans, almonds, seaweed, kelp, tea and meat.

Acupoints of Moxibustion

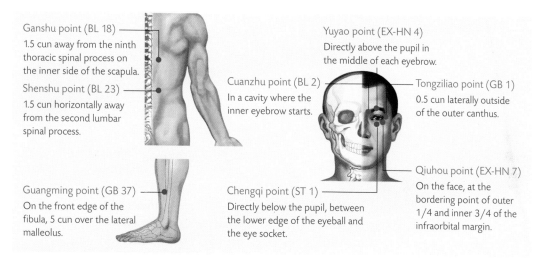

Ganshu point (BL 18)
1.5 cun away from the ninth thoracic spinal process on the inner side of the scapula.

Shenshu point (BL 23)
1.5 cun horizontally away from the second lumbar spinal process.

Yuyao point (EX-HN 4)
Directly above the pupil in the middle of each eyebrow.

Cuanzhu point (BL 2)
In a cavity where the inner eyebrow starts.

Tongziliao point (GB 1)
0.5 cun laterally outside of the outer canthus.

Qiuhou point (EX-HN 7)
On the face, at the bordering point of outer 1/4 and inner 3/4 of the infraorbital margin.

Guangming point (GB 37)
On the front edge of the fibula, 5 cun over the lateral malleolus.

Chengqi point (ST 1)
Directly below the pupil, between the lower edge of the eyeball and the eye socket.

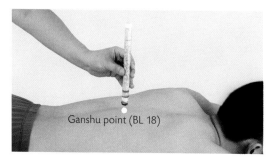

Ganshu point (BL 18)

Moxibustion Methods

Mild moxibustion: Moxibustion is applied to the Ganshu, Shenshu and Guangming points, starting with points on the upper body and then moving to those on the lower body. The patient should take an appropriate posture. The practitioner ignites a moxa roll at one end and points the ignited end at the points, 3 to 5 centimeters above the skin's surface, until the skin feels mildly warm without any burning pain. For a patient with decreased sensitivity, the practitioner can place the index finger and middle finger around the point to feel the temperature, so as not to burn patient's skin. Moxibustion lasts 5 to 10 minutes per point, until the skin turns slightly red. This moxibustion should be applied once or twice a day for 10 times as a course of treatment, with an interval of 3 to 5 days between two courses.

Swirling moxibustion: Moxibustion is applied to such points as Cuanzhu, Yuyao, Tongziliao, Chengqi and Qiuhou. The patient takes an appropriate posture. The practitioner ignites a moxa roll at one end and points the ignited end at the point about 3 centimeters above the skin's surface. The practitioner moves the moxa roll left and right or in a circle over the point, repeating the movement until the skin feels warm without any burning pain. The movement range is about 3 centimeters, and treatment will have no effect if the movement range is too large. Moxibustion lasts 10 minutes per point. This is performed once every day, for 10 times as a course of treatment, with an interval of 3 to 5 days between two courses.

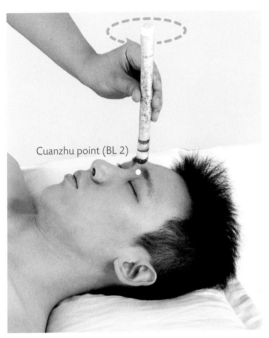

Cuanzhu point (BL 2)

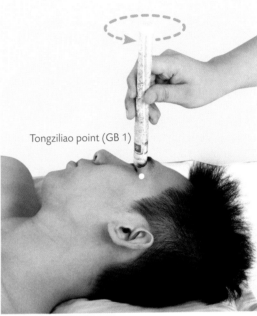

Tongziliao point (GB 1)

22. Shingles

Shingles is an acute inflammatory skin disease caused by varicella zoster virus. It is mainly characterized by blisters distributed in clusters along one side of the peripheral nerves and is often accompanied by obvious neuralgia. The disease often occurs in adults, most commonly in spring and autumn. Incidence increases significantly with age.

Moxibustion Method

Swirling moxibustion: Moxibustion is applied to such points as Jianzhen, Ganshu, Danshu, Waiguan, Xuehai, Ququan, Taichong, Xiaxi and Ashi, working from the upper to lower body. Patients are advised to perform moxibustion of the points within reach themselves in order to control the temperature.

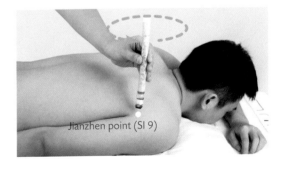

Jianzhen point (SI 9)

The patient should take an appropriate posture. The practitioner ignites a moxa roll at one end with the ignited end about 3 centimeters over the skin's surface, and moves near the point left and right, or circularly, within the range of about 3 centimeters. The temperature during moxibustion should make the patient feel warm without any burning pain. Apply moxibustion 20 to 30 minutes per point, until the local skin turns slightly red. Such treatment should be given once a day for a seven-day course of treatment, with an interval of three days between two courses.

Acupoints of Moxibustion

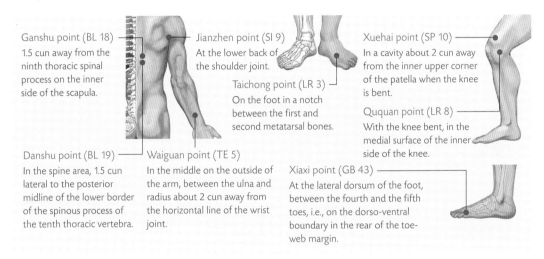

Ganshu point (BL 18)
1.5 cun away from the ninth thoracic spinal process on the inner side of the scapula.

Jianzhen point (SI 9)
At the lower back of the shoulder joint.

Taichong point (LR 3)
On the foot in a notch between the first and second metatarsal bones.

Xuehai point (SP 10)
In a cavity about 2 cun away from the inner upper corner of the patella when the knee is bent.

Ququan point (LR 8)
With the knee bent, in the medial surface of the inner side of the knee.

Danshu point (BL 19)
In the spine area, 1.5 cun lateral to the posterior midline of the lower border of the spinous process of the tenth thoracic vertebra.

Waiguan point (TE 5)
In the middle on the outside of the arm, between the ulna and radius about 2 cun away from the horizontal line of the wrist joint.

Xiaxi point (GB 43)
At the lateral dorsum of the foot, between the fourth and the fifth toes, i.e., on the dorso-ventral boundary in the rear of the toe-web margin.

23. Pruritus

Pruritus refers to a skin disease without a primary rash but with itching. Belonging to neuropsychiatric dermatosis, it is a neurosis of the skin and can be found all over the body or in local areas such as anus, scrotum or vulva. It is characterized by paroxysmal and intense itching, often aggravated at night, affecting sleep quality. Patients often scratch the affected area. Dry skin, exposure to pathogenic wind, insect infestation, mental stress, emotional fluctuation, and eating spicy food can all cause pruritus. Moxibustion at the relevant points can clear heat and expel dampness, dispel pathogenic wind and detoxify the body to reduce the symptoms of pruritus.

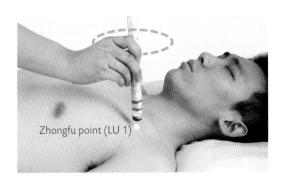

Zhongfu point (LU 1)

Moxibustion Method

Swirling moxibustion: Take two groups of points, one group consisting of Lieque, Fengmen, Feishu, Geshu and Pishu, and the other group consisting of Quchi, Zhongfu, Zhangmen and Fengshi. Choose one group of points in each moxibustion therapy. Perform moxibustion beginning with points on the waist and back and then moving on to the chest and abdomen, working from the upper to lower body. The patient should take an appropriate posture. The practitioner ignites a moxa roll, with the ignited end about 3 centimeters over the skin and targeting the acupoint. The practitioner holds the roll and moves it left and right or circularly, within a range of about 3 centimeters. Moxibustion lasts 20 to 30 minutes per point once a day for a seven-day course of treatment, with an interval of 3 to 5 days between two courses. The two groups of points should be used alternately.

Acupoints of Moxibustion

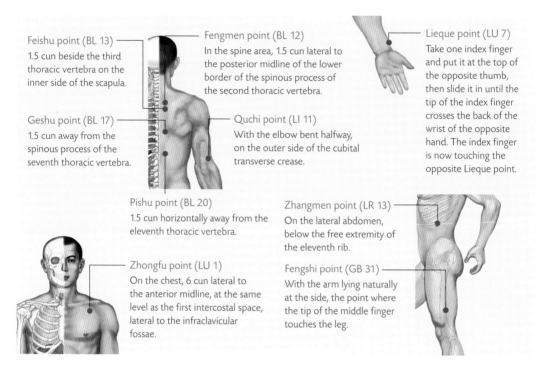

Feishu point (BL 13)
1.5 cun beside the third thoracic vertebra on the inner side of the scapula.

Fengmen point (BL 12)
In the spine area, 1.5 cun lateral to the posterior midline of the lower border of the spinous process of the second thoracic vertebra.

Lieque point (LU 7)
Take one index finger and put it at the top of the opposite thumb, then slide it in until the tip of the index finger crosses the back of the wrist of the opposite hand. The index finger is now touching the opposite Lieque point.

Geshu point (BL 17)
1.5 cun away from the spinous process of the seventh thoracic vertebra.

Quchi point (LI 11)
With the elbow bent halfway, on the outer side of the cubital transverse crease.

Pishu point (BL 20)
1.5 cun horizontally away from the eleventh thoracic vertebra.

Zhangmen point (LR 13)
On the lateral abdomen, below the free extremity of the eleventh rib.

Zhongfu point (LU 1)
On the chest, 6 cun lateral to the anterior midline, at the same level as the first intercostal space, lateral to the infraclavicular fossae.

Fengshi point (GB 31)
With the arm lying naturally at the side, the point where the tip of the middle finger touches the leg.

24. Hyperhidrosis

Hyperhidrosis is caused by hypersecretion of the eccrine gland and manifested by excessive systemic sweating in general hyperhidrosis or excessive local sweating in localized hyperhidrosis. Often occurring from early age, it is aggravated in adolescence and persists throughout the patient's life. In a severe case, it affects not only the patient's work, daily life and study, but also causes psychological problems and keeps patients from participating in normal social activities.

According to traditional Chinese medicine, endocrine disorders, physical weakness and mental factors can cause hyperhidrosis. Moxibustion on related points can regulate endocrine and improve physical resistance to diseases, thus relieving the symptoms.

To prevent and treat hyperhidrosis, one must first discover the cause. Patients should pay attention to hygiene, bathe frequently, change underwear and shoes and socks frequently, try to wear thin, soft, absorbent and breathable cotton products, avoiding underwear made of chemical fiber materials. The diet should be light, and patients should avoid eating spicy and irritating food. Keep peace of mind and a stable mood.

Acupoints of Moxibustion

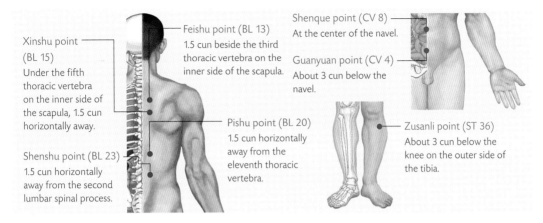

Xinshu point (BL 15)
Under the fifth thoracic vertebra on the inner side of the scapula, 1.5 cun horizontally away.

Feishu point (BL 13)
1.5 cun beside the third thoracic vertebra on the inner side of the scapula.

Shenshu point (BL 23)
1.5 cun horizontally away from the second lumbar spinal process.

Pishu point (BL 20)
1.5 cun horizontally away from the eleventh thoracic vertebra.

Shenque point (CV 8)
At the center of the navel.

Guanyuan point (CV 4)
About 3 cun below the navel.

Zusanli point (ST 36)
About 3 cun below the knee on the outer side of the tibia.

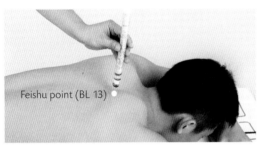

Feishu point (BL 13)

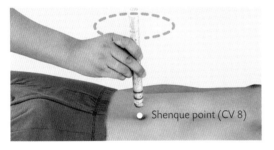

Shenque point (CV 8)

Moxibustion Methods

Mild moxibustion: Moxibustion is applied to the Feishu, Xinshu, Pishu, Shenshu and Zusanli points, beginning with the upper body and then moving to the lower body. The patient should take an appropriate posture. The practitioner ignites a moxa roll at one end and points the ignited end to a point, 3 to 5 centimeters above the skin's surface, until the patient's skin feels warm but without any burning pain. Moxibustion lasts 15 to 20 minutes for each point, until the skin turns slightly red. The treatment is given once or twice a day for 10 times as a course of treatment, with an interval of three days between two courses.

Swirling moxibustion: Moxibustion is applied to the Shenque and Guanyuan points. The patient should take a supine position, with the related skin area exposed. The practitioner ignites a moxa roll, and with the ignited end about 3 centimeters above the skin, moves it left and right or circularly, within the range of about 3 centimeters, until it brings mild warmth without the feeling of burning pain. Moxibustion lasts 10 to 15 minutes for each point, until the skin turns slightly red. This is performed once every day, for 10 times as a course of treatment, with an interval of 3 to 5 days between two courses.

The Soup of Black Bean, Longan and Chinese Dates

Ingredients: 1.1 ounces of black beans, 0.4 ounces of longan meat and 1.1 ounces of Chinese dates.

Preparation: Cook the soup with black beans, longan meat and Chinese dates. Eat twice a day for 15 days as a course of treatment. This soup is mainly for child hyperhidrosis, and those with sweating in their sleep, emaciated with cold limbs, and with dry mouth and dry stool.

25. Sciatica

Sciatica, a type of sciatic nerve lesions, refers to the pains within the range of the sciatic nerve, including the waist, buttocks, back of the thighs, posterior-lateral shanks and lateral feet. This disease is commonly seen in young men. In recent years, it has been particularly common among office workers and those who use computers for extended periods.

Patients should pay attention to diet, nutrition balance and daily life to help facilitate physical recovery. Take moderate physical exercise, paying attention to protecting the waist and affected limbs after exercise. Quit smoking and restrict drinking to enhance physical fitness and help lower the incidence of infection. Prevent the invasion of pathogenic wind, cold and damp, which can cause qi and blood stagnation and meridian obstruction. This is a contributing factor to both sciatica and aggravated sciatica. Develop good sitting, standing and sleeping postures, and adhere to scientific and reasonable health care methods.

Acupoints of Moxibustion

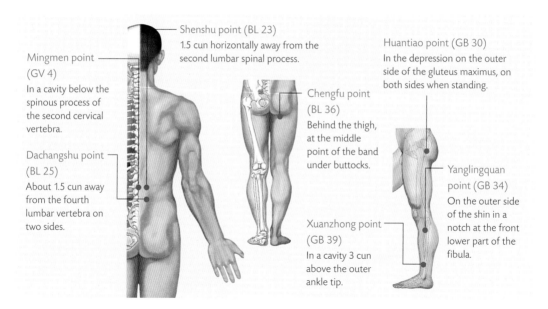

Shenshu point (BL 23)
1.5 cun horizontally away from the second lumbar spinal process.

Mingmen point (GV 4)
In a cavity below the spinous process of the second cervical vertebra.

Dachangshu point (BL 25)
About 1.5 cun away from the fourth lumbar vertebra on two sides.

Huantiao point (GB 30)
In the depression on the outer side of the gluteus maximus, on both sides when standing.

Chengfu point (BL 36)
Behind the thigh, at the middle point of the band under buttocks.

Yanglingquan point (GB 34)
On the outer side of the shin in a notch at the front lower part of the fibula.

Xuanzhong point (GB 39)
In a cavity 3 cun above the outer ankle tip.

Moxibustion Methods

Mild moxibustion: Moxibustion is applied to such points as Shenshu, Mingmen, Dachangshu, Huantiao, Chengfu, Yanglingquan and Xuanzhong, moving from points on the upper body to those on the lower body. The patient should take an appropriate posture. The practitioner, standing on one side of the patient, ignites a moxa roll at one end and points the ignited end at a point, 3 to 5 centimeters above the skin's surface, until the skin feels warm

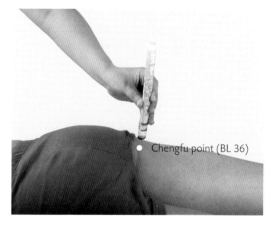

Chengfu point (BL 36)

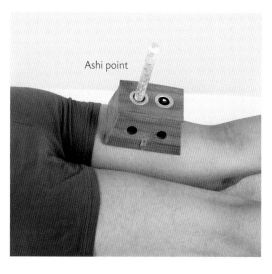
Ashi point

without burning pain. Moxibustion lasts 15 to 20 minutes for each point, until the local skin turns slightly red. Moxibustion should be applied once or twice a day for 10 times as a course of treatment, with an interval of 3 to 5 days between two courses. For a patient with decreased sensitivity, the practitioner can place an index finger and a middle finger around the point to feel the temperature and avoid burning the patient's skin.

Moxibustion with moxa stick roll holder: Moxibustion is applied to the Ashi point, i.e., the pain point. After the patient takes an appropriate posture, place the moxa stick roll holder on the Ashi point, ignite the moxa roll and put it on the mesh, and then close the cover to perform moxibustion. Moxibustion lasts 15 to 30 minutes for each point. This method is characterized by evenly distributed heat, which makes the patient feel comfortable. This is performed once or twice a day, for 10 times as a course of treatment, with an interval of 3 to 5 days between two courses.

The following exercises can complement moxibustion treatment. Consult a doctor for any unsuitable symptom before exercise.

1. Lifting legs: Take a supine posture, stretch lower limbs straight, lift the limbs up actively, and try to lift beyond your limit.

3. Forced exercise: Stand straight, flex the upper body forward and to the side and lift legs respectively.

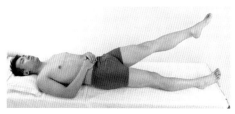

2. Rowing: Sit, straighten legs and flex the upper body forward, trying to touch the feet with hands each time, making a movement like rowing a boat.

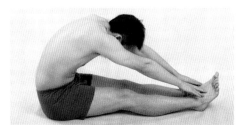

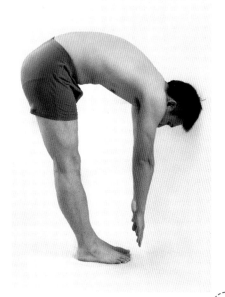

26. Stiff Neck

Stiff neck is an acute sprain or inflammation of the soft cervical tissue mainly manifested by neck pain, stiffness in the neck, and difficulty turning the head. Commonly there are no symptoms before going to sleep, but a sore neck and limited neck movement after getting up in the morning. This shows that this disease occurs after sleeping and has a close relationship with pillows and sleeping postures.

According to traditional Chinese medicine, poor sleeping posture, inappropriate pillows or cold may cause obstructed meridians, poor blood circulation, and stagnation of pathogenic cold in the neck. Moxibustion at relevant points can dredge meridians and expel pathogenic cold to treat a stiff neck.

Patients with frequent stiff necks should pay attention to the balance of their diets and should eat both meat and vegetables, as well as increase their intake of foods rich in vitamins and minerals such as fresh vegetables, fruits, dairy products and soy products. Choose comfortable pillows, avoid bad sleeping postures, avoid catching cold, catching a chill or getting wet in the rain. Keep the shoulders warm. Do a moderate amount of exercise and exercise the neck regularly.

Acupoints of Moxibustion

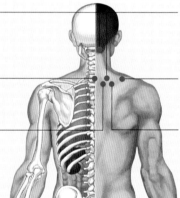

Tianzhu point (BL 10)
At the rear of the head, 1.5 cun from the middle line and 1 cun above the hairline.

Dazhui point (GV 14)
Under the spinous process of the seventh cervical vertebrae.

Dazhu point (BL 11)
In the spine area, 1.5 cun lateral to the posterior midline of the lower border of the spinous process of the first thoracic vertebra.

Jianzhongshu point (SI 15)
At the back, under the seventh spinous process of the cervical spine, 2 cun away from it.

Jianjing point (GB 21)
At the midpoint of the top on the shoulder.

Jianwaishu point (SI 14)
At the back, under the first spinous process of thoracic vertebra, 3 cun away from it.

Moxibustion Methods

Swirling moxibustion: Moxibustion is applied to such points as Dazhui, Jianjing and Dazhu. The patient takes a sitting or prone posture. The practitioner, standing on one side of the patient, ignites a moxa roll at one end and points the ignited end at a point, about 3 centimeters above the skin's surface. The practitioner holds and moves the roll left and right or circularly, within the range of about 3 centimeters, until the patient's skin feels warm, without any burning pain. Moxibustion lasts 10 to 15 minutes per

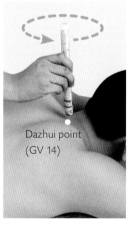

Dazhui point (GV 14)

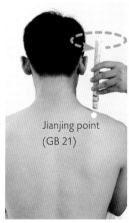

Jianjing point (GB 21)

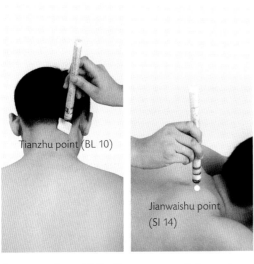

Tianzhu point (BL 10)

Jianwaishu point
(SI 14)

point, until the patient feels comfortable and the skin turns slightly red. This is performed once every day, and continued 1 to 3 more days after symptoms alleviate.

Mild moxibustion: Moxibustion is applied to the Dazhui, Tianzhu, Jianjing, Jianwaishu, Jianzhongshu points. The patient takes a sitting or prone posture. The practitioner ignites a moxa roll at one end and points the ignited end at a point, 3 to 5 centimeters above the skin's surface, until the patient's skin feels warm with no burning pain. For a patient with decreased sensitivity, the practitioner can place an index

finger and a middle finger around the point to feel the temperature and avoid burning the skin. Moxibustion lasts 15 to 20 minutes for each point, until the patient's skin turns slightly red. Such treatment should be given once or twice daily and continue 1 to 3 more days after symptoms alleviate. Place a slice of ginger on the point when performing moxibustion on the Tianzhu point to prevent falling ash from burning the hair.

27. Lumbar Disc Herniation

Lumbar disc herniation is a rupture of annulus fibrosus in the lumbar intervertebral disc and subsequent lumbar pain and numbness, caused by excessive fatigue, trauma or other factors. This frequently occurring orthopedic disease often occurs in young adults.

In the acute period, people with lumbar disc herniation should sleep on a hard bed and stay in bed for three weeks. Rehabilitation exercise is the key to the treatment of lumbar disc herniation. Patients with lumbar disc herniation should pay attention to dietary nutrition and eat more food with high protein and vitamin content, prevent obesity, quit smoking and control drinking. They should pay attention to the balance of work and rest, not sit or stand too long, and avoid heavy physical work. They should pay attention to keeping warm in cold and humid seasons.

Acupoints of Moxibustion

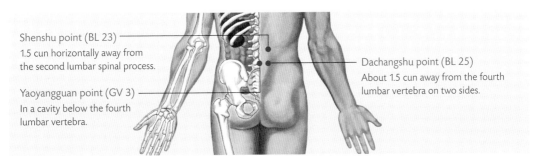

Shenshu point (BL 23)
1.5 cun horizontally away from the second lumbar spinal process.

Yaoyangguan point (GV 3)
In a cavity below the fourth lumbar vertebra.

Dachangshu point (BL 25)
About 1.5 cun away from the fourth lumbar vertebra on two sides.

Moxibustion Method

Mild moxibustion: Moxibustion is applied to such points as Shenshu, Dachangshu, Yaoyangguan and Ashi. The patient should take a prone posture. The practitioner stands on one side of the patient, ignites a moxa roll at one end and points it accurately at a point, 3 to 5 centimeters above the skin's surface, until the patient's skin feels warm, without the feeling of burning pain. For a patient with reduced sensitivity, the practitioner can place an index finger and a middle finger around the point to feel the temperature, so as not to burn the patient's skin. Moxibustion lasts 15 to 20 minutes per point, until the patient feels comfortable and the skin turns slightly red. This moxibustion

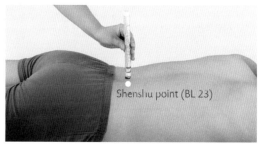
Shenshu point (BL 23)

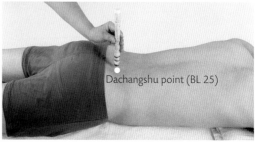
Dachangshu point (BL 25)

should be applied once or twice a day for 10 times as a course of treatment, with an interval of 1 to 3 days between two courses. During moxibustion, the practitioner should concentrate to avoid burning the skin with falling ash.

Simple massage also has an excellent effect on lumbar disc herniation. Gently press and knead the waist once a day. Two persons can massage the back of each other by carrying each other on the back alternately. Note that this method must be performed with caution, and no brute force should be exerted. Massage can activate the meridians, relax the muscles, and promote the circulation of qi and stop pain, thus relieving the symptoms.

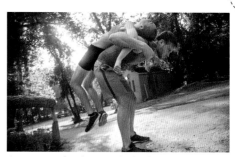
Carrying each other on the back.

28. Acute Lumbar Sprain

Acute lumbar sprain, commonly known as sudden lumbar sprain, is an acute sprain of soft lumbar tissues including muscles, ligaments, fascia and facet joints. Acute lumbar sprain is most common in young adults. It is mainly caused by weight-bearing beyond body's limit, improper posture, inharmonious movements, sudden slips, vigorous lifting, lack of preparation during activities and an overlarge range of activities.

Moxibustion Method

Mild moxibustion: Moxibustion is applied to such points as Shenshu, Dachangshu, Yaoyangguan and Ashi. The patient should take a prone posture, with related skin exposed.

The practitioner, standing on one side of the patient, ignites a moxa roll at one end and points the ignited end at a point, 3 to 5 centimeters above the skin's surface, until the patient's skin feels warm but without any burning pain. Moxibustion lasts 15 to 20 minutes per point, until the skin turns slightly red. This moxibustion should be applied once or twice a day for 10 times as a course of treatment, with an interval of 1 to 2 days between two courses.

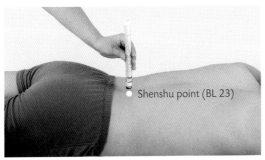
Shenshu point (BL 23)

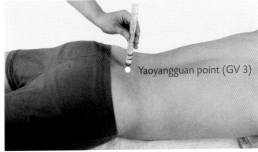
Yaoyangguan point (GV 3)

Acupoints of Moxibustion

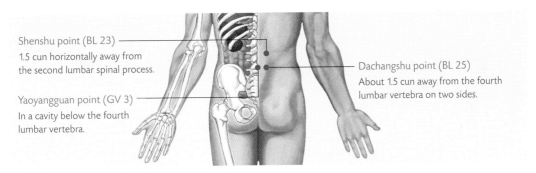

Shenshu point (BL 23)
1.5 cun horizontally away from the second lumbar spinal process.

Dachangshu point (BL 25)
About 1.5 cun away from the fourth lumbar vertebra on two sides.

Yaoyangguan point (GV 3)
In a cavity below the fourth lumbar vertebra.

29. Knee Osteoarthritis

Knee osteoarthritis refers to a chronic bone joint disease caused by the degeneration of the knee cartilage and bone hyperplasia. It can occur on one or both sides. It is more common among manual workers and overweight patients or those with high blood pressure.

According to traditional Chinese medicine, this disease is caused by exogenous pathogenic wind and deficiency of the liver and kidneys. Moxibustion at related points can benefit the liver and kidneys and expel pathogenic wind to relieve the symptoms.

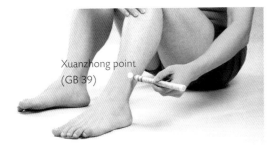
Xuanzhong point (GB 39)

Moxibustion Method

Sparrow-pecking moxibustion:
Moxibustion is applied to such points as Zusanli, Xuanzhong, Yanglingquan, Xuehai, Liangqiu and Ashi. Choose 3 to 6 of these points for each instance of treatment. Patients can perform moxibustion of accessible points themselves to control the

temperature. The patient takes an appropriate posture. The practitioner ignites a moxa roll at one end and points the ignited end at the point, about 3 centimeters above the skin's surface, and moves it up and down like a bird pecking at food. Avoid burning the skin with strong heat during treatment. The moxibustion should be given 10 to 15 minutes per point, once a day, for a 10-day for treatment course with a five-day interval between two courses.

Acupoints of Moxibustion

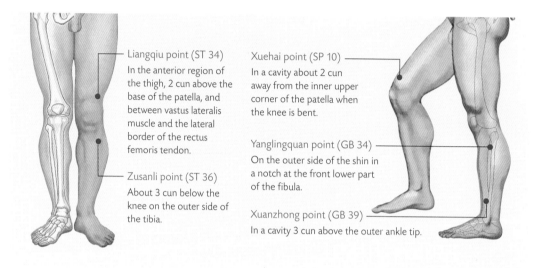

Liangqiu point (ST 34)
In the anterior region of the thigh, 2 cun above the base of the patella, and between vastus lateralis muscle and the lateral border of the rectus femoris tendon.

Zusanli point (ST 36)
About 3 cun below the knee on the outer side of the tibia.

Xuehai point (SP 10)
In a cavity about 2 cun away from the inner upper corner of the patella when the knee is bent.

Yanglingquan point (GB 34)
On the outer side of the shin in a notch at the front lower part of the fibula.

Xuanzhong point (GB 39)
In a cavity 3 cun above the outer ankle tip.

30. Ankle Sprain

Ankle sprain refers to tearing damage to the soft tissues around the joint, such as the joint capsule, ligament and tendon, when the joint suddenly moves to one side and exceeds its normal range of motion under the action of external force. Ankle sprain is a common type of injury, and can occur when walking, running, walking up and down the stairs or participating in sports. Moxibustion at the relevant points can improve blood circulation, relieve blood stasis, activate meridians, relax muscles, and relieve swelling and pain, thus improving symptoms.

Field first aid for an ankle sprain: Stop the activity and loosen the shoelace or take off the shoes immediately after the sprain; apply a cold compress to the wounded area or soak the affected area in cold water for 20 to 30 minutes to help eliminate the pain. Do not massage the affected area with the hands; go to the hospital to examine for fractures before treating.

Moxibustion Method

Mild moxibustion: Moxibustion is applied to the Jiexi and Ashi points. The patient takes an appropriate posture. The practitioner ignites a moxa roll at one end and points the ignited end at a point, 3 to 5 centimeters

Acupoints of Moxibustion

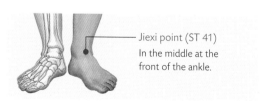

Jiexi point (ST 41)
In the middle at the front of the ankle.

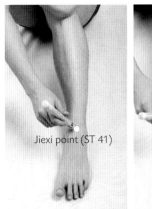

Jiexi point (ST 41)

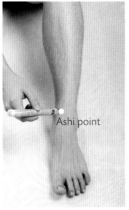

Ashi point

above the skin's surface, until the patient's skin feels warm, without the feeling of burning pain. For a patient with decreased sensitivity, the practitioner can place an index finger and a middle finger around the point to feel the temperature and avoid burning the skin. Moxibustion lasts 15 to 20 minutes per point, until the patient's local skin turns slightly red. This moxibustion should be applied once or twice a day for seven times as a course of treatment, with an interval of 1 to 2 days between two courses.

Ankle sprains are divided into inversion ankle sprains and eversion ankle sprains. Attention should be paid to the type of sprains to treat them differently. After the swelling following the sprain has subsided, simple massage can be performed to promote blood circulation, dissolve stasis and activate meridians. Massage can be performed to the shanks and local skin to ease the muscles, for about five minutes, once a day.

31. Hemorrhoids

Hemorrhoids include internal hemorrhoids, external hemorrhoids and mixed hemorrhoids. This is a chronic disease in which the anorectal bottom and venous plexus of anal mucosa develop varicose veins and form one or more soft venous masses. The common symptoms are pain in the affected area, blood in the excrement, etc. There are many causes, mainly including irregular daily life, sitting and standing for a long time, tiredness, constipation and pregnancy.

Acupoints of Moxibustion

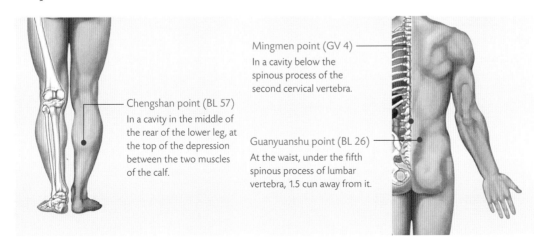

Mingmen point (GV 4)
In a cavity below the spinous process of the second cervical vertebra.

Chengshan point (BL 57)
In a cavity in the middle of the rear of the lower leg, at the top of the depression between the two muscles of the calf.

Guanyuanshu point (BL 26)
At the waist, under the fifth spinous process of lumbar vertebra, 1.5 cun away from it.

Moxibustion Method

Mild moxibustion: Moxibustion is applied to the Chengshan, Guanyuanshu and Mingmen points, moving from the upper to lower body. The patient takes an appropriate posture. The practitioner ignites a moxa roll at one end and points the ignited end at a point, 3 to 5 centimeters above the skin's surface, until the skin feels warm, without the feeling of burning pain. Moxibustion is performed for 10 minutes at each point, until the skin turns slightly red. Treatment should be given once a day for a 10-day course of treatment with an one-day interval between two courses.

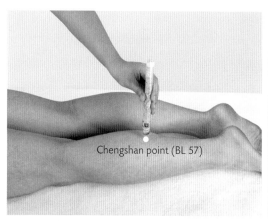

Chengshan point (BL 57)

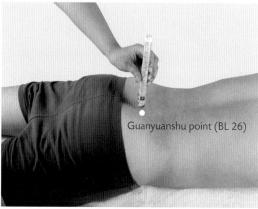

Guanyuanshu point (BL 26)

32. Chronic Appendicitis

Chronic appendicitis refers to the chronic inflammatory lesions of the appendix left behind after the acute inflammation of the appendix disappears, and can include fibrous connective tissue proliferation, stenosis or occlusion of the lumen, distortion of the appendix, and adhesion to surrounding tissues. The main symptoms are pressing abdominal pain, indigestion and emaciation. Moxibustion has an anti-inflammatory effect, and moxibustion at relevant points can eliminate inflammation, thus effectively treating chronic appendicitis.

Moxibustion Method

Mild moxibustion: Moxibustion is applied to such points as Yanglingquan, Qimen, Danshu and Taichong, plus Dazhui and Hegu points for patients with fever, and Qiuxu and Zusanli points for patients with colic pain. The moxibustion should be performed beginning with points on the waist and back and then moving on to those on the chest and abdomen, and working from the upper to lower body. The patient should take an appropriate position. The practitioner ignites one end of a moxa roll

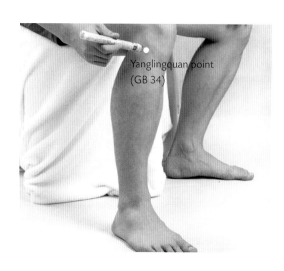

Yanglingquan point (GB 34)

and points the ignited end at a point, 3 to 5 centimeters above the skin's surface, until the patient feels warmth without burning pain. Moxibustion lasts 15 to 20 minutes for each point, until the skin surrounding the point turns slightly red. Such treatment should be given once a day and repeated 10 times for a course of treatment with at an interval of 1 to 2 days between two courses.

Acupoints of Moxibustion

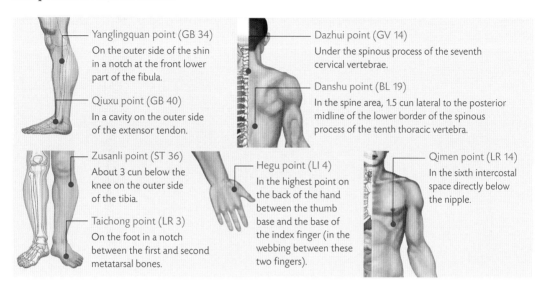

Yanglingquan point (GB 34)
On the outer side of the shin in a notch at the front lower part of the fibula.

Qiuxu point (GB 40)
In a cavity on the outer side of the extensor tendon.

Zusanli point (ST 36)
About 3 cun below the knee on the outer side of the tibia.

Taichong point (LR 3)
On the foot in a notch between the first and second metatarsal bones.

Hegu point (LI 4)
In the highest point on the back of the hand between the thumb base and the base of the index finger (in the webbing between these two fingers).

Dazhui point (GV 14)
Under the spinous process of the seventh cervical vertebrae.

Danshu point (BL 19)
In the spine area, 1.5 cun lateral to the posterior midline of the lower border of the spinous process of the tenth thoracic vertebra.

Qimen point (LR 14)
In the sixth intercostal space directly below the nipple.

33. Prolapse of the Anus

Prolapse of the anus, also known as rectal prolapse, is a phenomenon in which part or all of the rectal wall slides out of place and sometimes protrudes from the anus. In mild cases, the rectal mucosa prolapses during bowel movements, then can retract spontaneously; in severe cases, the rectum prolapses completely. Besides during bowel movements, it prolapses even during coughing, walking and squatting, and must be pushed back with the hands or will retract only after bed rest.

The occurrence of prolapse of the anus is related to many factors, and we must actively prevent it. Immediately treat diseases that can cause rectal prolapse, such as chronic diarrhea and constipation. Eat more vegetables and fruits, eat less spicy and irritating food like peppers and wine. Maintain smooth excrement. Keep the anus clean. It is recommended to wash the anus with warm water before going to bed, which can not only keep it clean, but also promote blood circulation in the anus. Develop a good habit of defecation. Do not read books or newspapers during defecation, and do not defecate with excessive force.

Moxibustion Method

Mild moxibustion: Moxibustion is applied to the Baihui point. The patient should take a sitting posture. The practitioner, standing on one side of the patient, ignites a moxa roll at one end and points the ignited end at a point, 3 to 5 centimeters above the skin's surface, until the patient feels warmth without the feeling of burning pain. Treatment is generally applied 15 to 20 minutes per point. This is performed once or twice a day, for 10 times as a course of treatment, with an interval of 3 to 5 days between two courses. During moxibustion of the Baihui point, the hair at the point should be parted to both sides before moxibustion or a slice of ginger placed on the point to avoid burning the hair.

Acupoint of Moxibustion

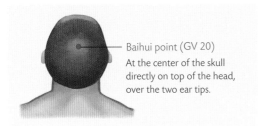

Baihui point (GV 20)
At the center of the skull directly on top of the head, over the two ear tips.

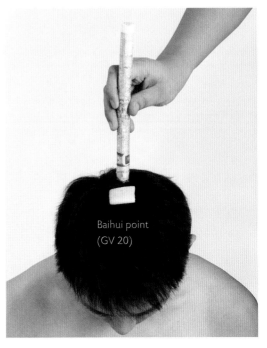

Baihui point
(GV 20)

Sea Cucumber Lean Meat Soup
Ingredients: 1.1 ounces of sea cucumber, appropriate amount of lean meat.
　　Preparation: Add an appropriate amount of water to the sea cucumber and lean meat to cook the soup; add salt for seasoning before eating. This soup serves to warm up yang, benefit qi and raise the anus.

34. Dysmenorrhea

Dysmenorrhea is a common gynecological disease. Symptoms are lower abdomen or lower back pain and even pain in the lumbosacral spine during and after menstruation. It attacks during each menstrual period. In severe cases, it may be accompanied by nausea and vomiting, incessant cold sweat, cold hands and feet, and even fainting, affecting work and life.
　　According to traditional Chinese medicine, dysmenorrhea is caused by qi and blood stagnation, stagnancy of cold and dampness, physical weakness, and liver and kidneys deficiency. Moxibustion at the relevant points can regulate qi and blood, expel dampness and cold, and invigorate the liver and kidneys, thereby reducing the symptoms of dysmenorrhea.

Moxibustion Methods

Mild moxibustion: Moxibustion is applied to such points as Qihai, Zhongji, Xuehai, Sanyinjiao and Xingjian, working from the upper to lower body. The patient should take an appropriate posture. The practitioner, standing on one side of the patient, ignites a moxa roll at one end and points the ignited end at a point, 3 to 5 centimeters above the skin's surface,

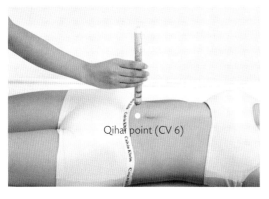

Qihai point (CV 6)

until the patient's skin feels warmth without burning pain. Moxibustion lasts 10 to 15 minutes for each point, until the skin turns slightly red. It is performed once or twice a day, for three times as a course of treatment, with an interval of two days between two courses. This method should be performed between two menstrual periods. It is suitable for dysmenorrhea caused by qi stagnation, which is marked by aggravation when the patient feels unhappy. Before menstruation, she may feel agitated with stuffiness in the chest and might fly into a rage over trifles; these symptoms are coupled with distension in breasts, the chest and ribs.

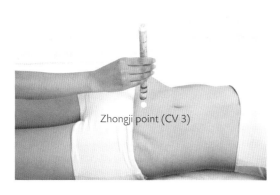

Zhongji point (CV 3)

Mild moxibustion: Moxibustion is applied to such points as Ciliao, Zhongji, Shuidao, Zigong and Diji, treating first the points on the waist and back and then those on the chest and abdomen, moving from the upper to the lower body. The patient should take an appropriate posture. The practitioner ignites one end of a moxa roll and points it at an acupoint, with the ignited end 3 to 5 centimeters above the skin's surface, until the patient feels warmth, without the feeling of burning pain. Moxibustion lasts 10 to 15 minutes for each point, until the skin turns slightly red. The method should be used between two menstrual periods. It is performed once or twice a day, for three times as a course of treatment, with an interval of two days between two courses. This treats dysmenorrhea caused by cold and dampness stagnation, which is characterized by aggravation in cold and damp situations. The lower abdomen feels comfortable with warmth and pressure. Warmth can reduce pain and the symptom of light-colored and sparse menstrual blood, as well as sore waist, weak legs, cold hands and feet, and also clear and abundant urine.

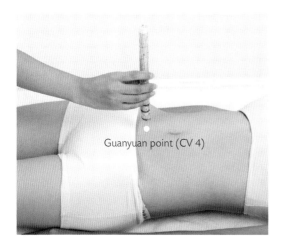

Guanyuan point (CV 4)

Mild moxibustion: Moxibustion is applied to such points as Ganshu, Pishu, Shenshu, Guanyuan, Mingmen, Ciliao, Shuidao, Zigong, Xuehai, Zusanli and Sanyinjiao, beginning with points on the waist and back and then moving on to those on the chest and abdomen, working from the upper to lower body. The patient should take an appropriate posture. The practitioner ignites one end of a moxa roll and points the ignited end at a point, 3 to 5 centimeters above the skin's surface, until the patient's skin feels warmth but not any burning pain. Moxibustion is performed 10 to 20 minutes for each point, once or twice a day. This is performed between two menstrual periods, for three times as a course of treatment, with an interval of two days between two courses. This is for dysmenorrhea caused by deficiency of qi and blood, which is manifested as dull pain in the lower abdomen, which feels hollow when pressed. The blood of menstruation looks light-colored and thin in small amount, coupled with pale and sallow complexion and low spirits.

Acupoints of Moxibustion

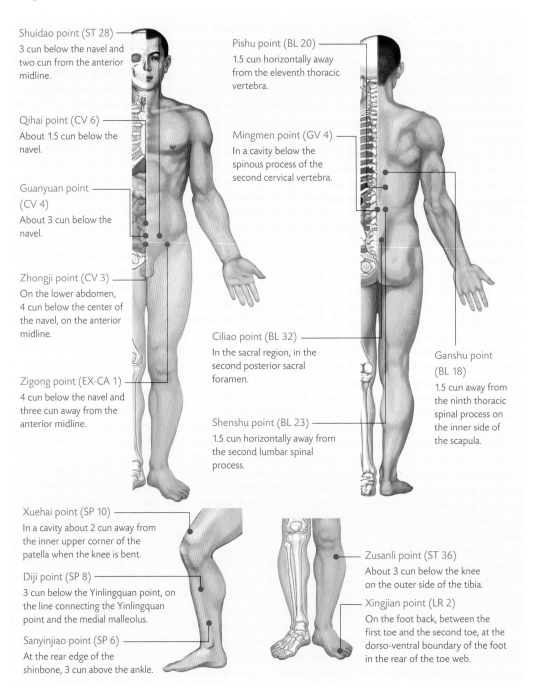

Shuidao point (ST 28)
3 cun below the navel and two cun from the anterior midline.

Qihai point (CV 6)
About 1.5 cun below the navel.

Guanyuan point
(CV 4)
About 3 cun below the navel.

Zhongji point (CV 3)
On the lower abdomen, 4 cun below the center of the navel, on the anterior midline.

Zigong point (EX-CA 1)
4 cun below the navel and three cun away from the anterior midline.

Pishu point (BL 20)
1.5 cun horizontally away from the eleventh thoracic vertebra.

Mingmen point (GV 4)
In a cavity below the spinous process of the second cervical vertebra.

Ciliao point (BL 32)
In the sacral region, in the second posterior sacral foramen.

Shenshu point (BL 23)
1.5 cun horizontally away from the second lumbar spinal process.

Ganshu point
(BL 18)
1.5 cun away from the ninth thoracic spinal process on the inner side of the scapula.

Xuehai point (SP 10)
In a cavity about 2 cun away from the inner upper corner of the patella when the knee is bent.

Diji point (SP 8)
3 cun below the Yinlingquan point, on the line connecting the Yinlingquan point and the medial malleolus.

Sanyinjiao point (SP 6)
At the rear edge of the shinbone, 3 cun above the ankle.

Zusanli point (ST 36)
About 3 cun below the knee on the outer side of the tibia.

Xingjian point (LR 2)
On the foot back, between the first toe and the second toe, at the dorso-ventral boundary of the foot in the rear of the toe web.

35. Amenorrhea

Amenorrhea refers to a condition in which a woman of over 18 years of age has no menstrual discharge or experiences a sudden nonphysiological interruption to menstruation of more than three months, when a normal menstrual cycle has already been established. Amenorrhea is related to systemic diseases, endocrine disorders, mental factors, and diseases such as severe anemia, tuberculosis, kidney disease and heart disease.

   There are many causes for amenorrhea. In addition to identifying the reasons and necessary treatment, one should also follow certain principles in diet. Those with weak constitutions should eat more nutritious and tonic food that can replenish and invigorate the blood and meridians, such as eggs, milk, Chinese dates, longan, walnuts and mutton. For amenorrhea caused by qi and blood stagnation, eat more food effective in invigorating blood and dissolving the stagnant, like ginger, Chinese dates and brown sugar. Patients can also decoct and drink brown sugar water daily. Patients must not only have comprehensive nutrition, but also exercise properly to enhance physical fitness and keep a positive outlook about treatment of the disease.

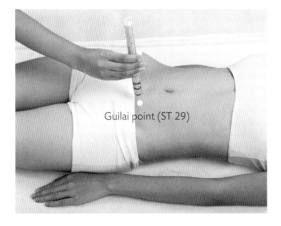

Guilai point (ST 29)

Moxibustion Method

Mild moxibustion: Moxibustion is applied to such points as Geshu, Ganshu, Shenshu, Pishu, Qihai, Guanyuan, Guilai, Zusanli and Sanyinjiao, beginning with points on the waist and back and then moving to those on the chest and abdomen, working from the upper to lower body. The patient should take an appropriate posture. The practitioner ignites one end of a moxa roll and points the ignited end at a point, 3 to 5 centimeters above the skin's surface, until the patient feels warm, without the feeling of burning pain. Moxibustion lasts 10 to 15 minutes for each point, until the skin turns slightly red. This is performed once a day and 15 sessions makes a course of treatment with an interval of 3 to 5 days between two courses.

Acupoints of Moxibustion

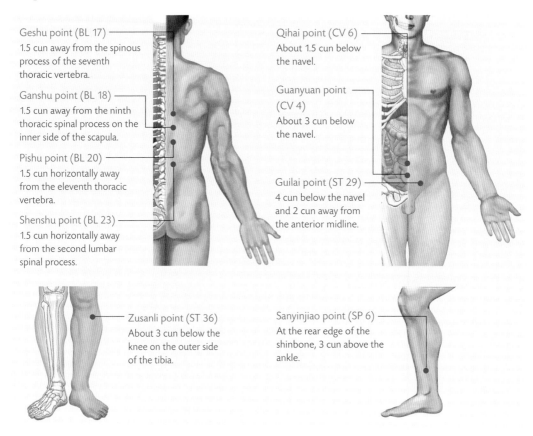

Geshu point (BL 17)
1.5 cun away from the spinous process of the seventh thoracic vertebra.

Ganshu point (BL 18)
1.5 cun away from the ninth thoracic spinal process on the inner side of the scapula.

Pishu point (BL 20)
1.5 cun horizontally away from the eleventh thoracic vertebra.

Shenshu point (BL 23)
1.5 cun horizontally away from the second lumbar spinal process.

Qihai point (CV 6)
About 1.5 cun below the navel.

Guanyuan point (CV 4)
About 3 cun below the navel.

Guilai point (ST 29)
4 cun below the navel and 2 cun away from the anterior midline.

Zusanli point (ST 36)
About 3 cun below the knee on the outer side of the tibia.

Sanyinjiao point (SP 6)
At the rear edge of the shinbone, 3 cun above the ankle.

36. Chronic Pelvic Inflammation

Chronic pelvic inflammatory disease refers to chronic inflammation of the female genitalia and its surrounding connective tissue and pelvic peritoneum. The main clinical manifestations are menstrual disorders, increased leucorrhea, lumbar and abdominal pain, and infertility. If chronic annexitis has been established, a lump can be felt.

Patients with pelvic inflammatory disease should pay attention to regulating diet. They should eat high-protein and high-vitamin food, like lean meat, tofu, chicken, fruits and vegetables. They should not eat spicy or irritating food, such as pepper, wine or strong tea. They should pay attention to personal hygiene and wash the genitals with water every day to prevent various infections. At the same time, they should also pay attention to contraception and control sexual activity; in addition, appropriate physical exercise can enhance physical fitness and promote recovery speed. Keeping a positive attitude is helpful for treatment.

Acupoints of Moxibustion

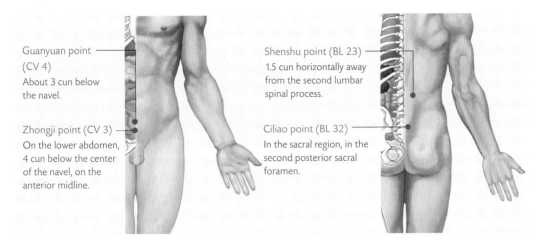

Guanyuan point (CV 4)
About 3 cun below the navel.

Zhongji point (CV 3)
On the lower abdomen, 4 cun below the center of the navel, on the anterior midline.

Shenshu point (BL 23)
1.5 cun horizontally away from the second lumbar spinal process.

Ciliao point (BL 32)
In the sacral region, in the second posterior sacral foramen.

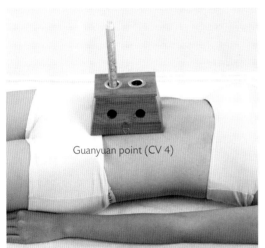

Guanyuan point (CV 4)

Moxibustion Method

Moxibustion with moxa stick roll holder: Moxibustion is applied to such points as Guanyuan, Zhongji, Shenshu and Ciliao, beginning with the points on the waist and back and then moving on to those on the chest and abdomen. The patient should take an appropriate posture. Choose a large-sized moxa stick roll holder and place it on the points for moxibustion. Ignite a moxa roll and put it on the mesh, then close the cover to perform moxibustion. Moxibustion lasts 15 to 30 minutes for each point. It is performed once or twice a day, for 10 times as a course of treatment, with an interval of 3 to 5 days between two courses. This therapy is characterized by evenly distributed heat, which makes the patient feel comfortable.

37. Pruritus Vulvae

Pruritus vulvae refers to a kind of subjective symptom caused by various vulvar lesions, and can occur in people with completely normal vulvae. The itchiness is mostly located at the clitoris and labia minora and can also affect the labia majora, perineum, and the perianal area. The attack can be paroxysmal and persistent, is often worst at night.

Diet regulation and eating light, vitamin-rich fresh vegetables and soy products can help prevent and treat pruritus vulvae. Avoid alcohol, coffee, strong tea, pepper and other irritating foods. Keep bowel movements smooth and prevent constipation. Keep underwear clean and change the underwear daily; also clean the genitals every day. Do not scratch when itching occurs, as scratches can aggravate itching and form a vicious circle. Staying positive can help the treatment work.

Moxibustion Method

Mild moxibustion: Moxibustion is applied to the Qihaishu, Zhonglushu, Dachangshu, Zhongji, Yinlian, Xuehai, Sanyinjiao, Yinjiao and Taixi points, beginning with points on the waist and back and moving on to those on the chest and abdomen, working from the upper to lower body. The patient should take an appropriate position. The practitioner ignites a moxa roll at one end and points

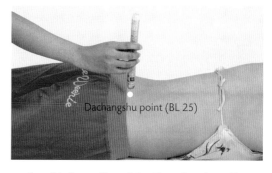

Dachangshu point (BL 25)

the ignited end at a point, 3 to 5 centimeters above the skin's surface. Moxibustion lasts 5 to 10 minutes for each point, until the patient feels comfortable and the skin turns slightly red. Such treatment should be given once daily for a 15-day course of treatment with an interval of three days between two courses. This therapy is the most suitable for genital itching caused by yin deficiency of the liver and kidneys.

Acupoints of Moxibustion

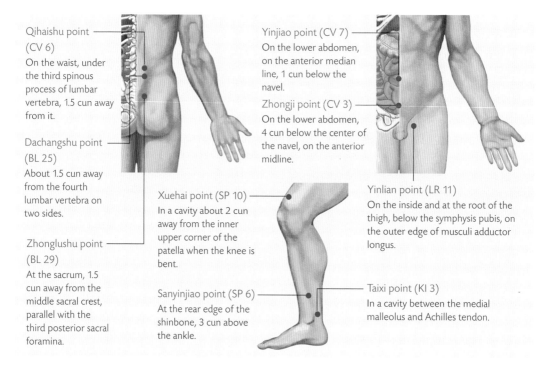

Qihaishu point (CV 6)
On the waist, under the third spinous process of lumbar vertebra, 1.5 cun away from it.

Dachangshu point (BL 25)
About 1.5 cun away from the fourth lumbar vertebra on two sides.

Zhonglushu point (BL 29)
At the sacrum, 1.5 cun away from the middle sacral crest, parallel with the third posterior sacral foramina.

Xuehai point (SP 10)
In a cavity about 2 cun away from the inner upper corner of the patella when the knee is bent.

Sanyinjiao point (SP 6)
At the rear edge of the shinbone, 3 cun above the ankle.

Yinjiao point (CV 7)
On the lower abdomen, on the anterior median line, 1 cun below the navel.

Zhongji point (CV 3)
On the lower abdomen, 4 cun below the center of the navel, on the anterior midline.

Yinlian point (LR 11)
On the inside and at the root of the thigh, below the symphysis pubis, on the outer edge of musculi adductor longus.

Taixi point (KI 3)
In a cavity between the medial malleolus and Achilles tendon.

Kelp and Bean Porridge
Ingredients: 3.5 ounces of rice, 1.1 ounces of kelp, 1.1 ounces of green beans, appropriate amount of sugar.

    Preparation: First wash and chop the kelp, soak green beans for half a day, wash rice clean, and combine all three ingredients to cook the porridge. Add white sugar when the porridge is soft and well-cooked. Eat the dish every morning and evening for 7 to 10 days. It can clear away heat, detoxify the body and help promote urination. This therapy is for relieving pruritus vulvae.

38. Female Sexual Dysfunction

This refers to persistent, recurrent problems with sexual response, desire or orgasm, which distress the patient or strain patients's relationship with her partner. Female sexual dysfunction can have physical and psychological causes. Moxibustion at related points can clear the liver and regulate qi, promote blood circulation, and nourish kidneys and yin, hence effectively improving the condition.

Acupoints of Moxibustion

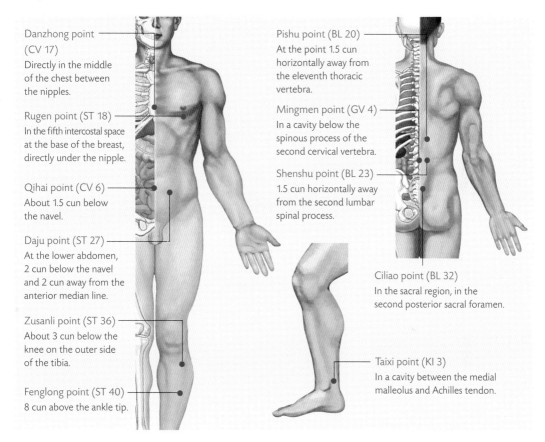

Danzhong point (CV 17)
Directly in the middle of the chest between the nipples.

Rugen point (ST 18)
In the fifth intercostal space at the base of the breast, directly under the nipple.

Qihai point (CV 6)
About 1.5 cun below the navel.

Daju point (ST 27)
At the lower abdomen, 2 cun below the navel and 2 cun away from the anterior median line.

Zusanli point (ST 36)
About 3 cun below the knee on the outer side of the tibia.

Fenglong point (ST 40)
8 cun above the ankle tip.

Pishu point (BL 20)
At the point 1.5 cun horizontally away from the eleventh thoracic vertebra.

Mingmen point (GV 4)
In a cavity below the spinous process of the second cervical vertebra.

Shenshu point (BL 23)
1.5 cun horizontally away from the second lumbar spinal process.

Ciliao point (BL 32)
In the sacral region, in the second posterior sacral foramen.

Taixi point (KI 3)
In a cavity between the medial malleolus and Achilles tendon.

Moxibustion Methods

Mild moxibustion: Moxibustion is applied to the Daju, Danzhong, Rugen, Qihai, Ciliao, Mingmen, Shenshu, Taixi, Pishu and Zusanli points, beginning with points on the waist and back and then moving on to those on chest and abdomen, working from the upper to lower body. The patient should take an appropriate posture. The practitioner, standing on one side of the patient, ignites a moxa roll at one end and points the ignited end at a point, 3 to 5 centimeters above the skin's surface, until the patient feels warm, without the feeling of burning pain. Moxibustion lasts 15 minutes at each point and is given once a day for a 10-day course of treatment, with a three-day interval between two courses. This therapy is the most suitable for female sexual dysfunction caused by deficiency syndrome (referring to a person with weakness of vital-qi due to congenital deficiency or acquired malnutrition). Symptoms are low libido and aversion to sex, accompanied by cold limbs, cold in the lower abdomen, occasional amenorrhea, lusterless complexion, insomnia, forgetfulness, and soreness and weakness of the waist and knees.

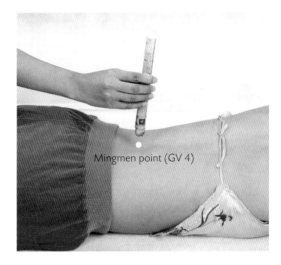
Mingmen point (GV 4)

Mild moxibustion: Moxibustion is applied to the Daju, Danzhong, Rugen, Qihai, Ciliao, Mingmen and Fenglong points, beginning with the waist and back and then moving to the chest and abdomen, working from the upper to lower body. The patient should take an appropriate posture. The practitioner holds a moxa roll, ignites one end and points the ignited end at a point, 3 to 5 centimeters above the skin's surface, until the patient feels warmth but no pain. Moxibustion lasts 15 minutes for each point and should be given once daily for a 10-day course of treatment with a three-day interval between two courses. This therapy is most suitable for frigidity caused by pathogenic phlegm-damp. Its main symptoms are low libido and aversion to sex, accompanied by physical obesity, loss of appetite, heaviness in the limbs, and thick leucorrhea.

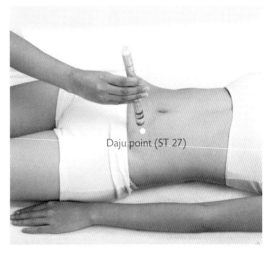
Daju point (ST 27)

39. Female Infertility

Infertility is diagnosed in a couple if they have normal reproductive functions and take no contraceptive measures but are unable to conceive after a year of normal sexual activity. There are many reasons for female infertility. One is the inability to ovulate, and another is infertility due to the eggs and sperm not joining. These two issues may or may not be reversible.

There are many causes of female infertility, including disorder of the reproductive system, recurrent miscarriage, and various gynecological diseases. However, most cases of infertility can be prevented. All kinds of gynecological diseases affecting pregnancy, such as menstruation and morbid leucorrhea, especially gynecological inflammation, dysmenorrhea, amenorrhea, uterine bleeding, and irregular menstruation, must be promptly regulated and treated. Avoid recurrent medical or surgical abortion to prevent secondary infertility or habitual abortion. It is necessary to treat infertility correctly, reduce psychological pressure and remain positive to enhance the chance of conception.

Acupoints of Moxibustion

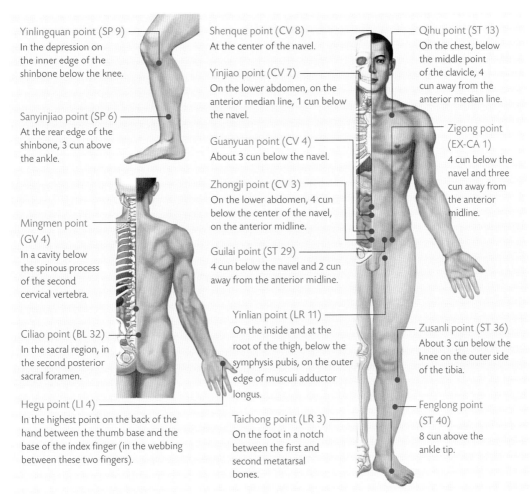

Yinlingquan point (SP 9)
In the depression on the inner edge of the shinbone below the knee.

Sanyinjiao point (SP 6)
At the rear edge of the shinbone, 3 cun above the ankle.

Mingmen point (GV 4)
In a cavity below the spinous process of the second cervical vertebra.

Ciliao point (BL 32)
In the sacral region, in the second posterior sacral foramen.

Hegu point (LI 4)
In the highest point on the back of the hand between the thumb base and the base of the index finger (in the webbing between these two fingers).

Shenque point (CV 8)
At the center of the navel.

Yinjiao point (CV 7)
On the lower abdomen, on the anterior median line, 1 cun below the navel.

Guanyuan point (CV 4)
About 3 cun below the navel.

Zhongji point (CV 3)
On the lower abdomen, 4 cun below the center of the navel, on the anterior midline.

Guilai point (ST 29)
4 cun below the navel and 2 cun away from the anterior midline.

Yinlian point (LR 11)
On the inside and at the root of the thigh, below the symphysis pubis, on the outer edge of musculi adductor longus.

Taichong point (LR 3)
On the foot in a notch between the first and second metatarsal bones.

Qihu point (ST 13)
On the chest, below the middle point of the clavicle, 4 cun away from the anterior median line.

Zigong point (EX-CA 1)
4 cun below the navel and three cun away from the anterior midline.

Zusanli point (ST 36)
About 3 cun below the knee on the outer side of the tibia.

Fenglong point (ST 40)
8 cun above the ankle tip.

Moxibustion Methods

Mild moxibustion: Moxibustion is applied to such points as Mingmen, Qihu, Shenque, Yinjiao, Guanyuan, Zhongji, Zigong, Zusanli and Sanyinjiao, beginning with points on the waist and back and then moving on to those on the chest and abdomen, working from the upper to lower body. The patient should take an appropriate posture, with the related skin areas exposed. The practitioner ignites a moxa roll at one end and points the ignited end at a point, 3 to 5 centimeters above the skin's surface, until the patient feels warm, without the feeling of burning pain. Moxibustion lasts 15 to 20 minutes for each point, until the skin turns red. This should be performed once a day for a 10-day course of treatment with an interval of 3 to 5 days between two courses. This therapy is most suitable for patients with infertility due to deficiency of the kidneys, cold womb and deficiency of blood.

Patients with kidney deficiency usually experience dizziness, tinnitus, soreness and weakness of waist and knees, decline of sexual functions, and for men, small amount of sperm and frequent occurrence of spermatorrhea. Women experiencing infertility sometimes also experience early exhaustion of menstruation, early aging, low spirits, forgetfulness, frequent urination in the daytime, remaining urine after urine is discharged, clear and abundant urine at night and urinary incontinence along with light tongue surface and a little tongue coating.

The so-called cold womb refers to the deficiency of kidney yang and the absence of warmth in the womb, hence leading to distension and pain in the lower abdomen, which can be relieved by applying warmth, as well as lots of leucorrhea, dysmenorrhea, irregular menstruation, thin white tongue coating, and excess saliva.

Deficiency of blood refers to malnutrition of the inner organs, meridians and the body, commonly characterized by pale or sallow complexion, dizziness, poor eyesight, palpitations, more dreams, numb hands and feet, menstruation in a small amount with light color, and pale lips, tongue and nails. In the late period, patients might encounter amenorrhea and a weak pulse.

Mild moxibustion: Moxibustion is applied to such points as Zhongji, Hegu, Sanyinjiao, Qihu, Yinlian, Yinlingquan, Fenglong, Guilai, Ciliao, Zigong and Taichong, moving from the points on the waist and back to those on the chest and abdomen, working from the upper to lower body. The patient takes an appropriate posture. The practitioner ignites a moxa roll at one end and points the ignited end at a point, 3 to 5 centimeters above the skin's surface, until the patient feels warmth at the point, without burning pain. Moxibustion lasts 15 to 20 minutes for each point, until the patient feels comfortable and the skin turns red. This should be performed once a day for a 10-day course of treatment with an interval of 3 to 5 days between two courses. This therapy is most suitable for patients with infertility due to stagnation of qi, obstruction of phlegm, and blood stasis in uterine collaterals, with symptoms of cold hands and feet, prickling pain in the lower abdomen, and fear of being touched and pressed, in addition to a fat tongue, sticky white tongue coating, a gray or spotted tongue and irregular menstruation.

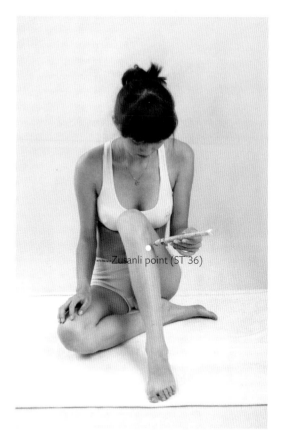

Zusanli point (ST 36)

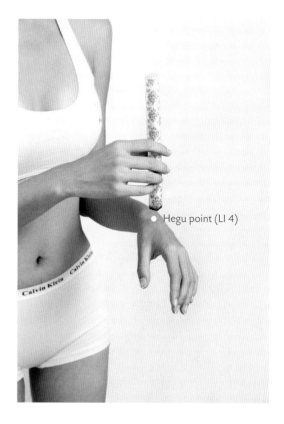

Hegu point (LI 4)

Leek Fried Shrimps

Ingredients: 8.8 ounces of shrimps, 3.5 ounces of leeks, appropriate amount of yellow rice wine, soy sauce, vinegar and ginger slices.

Preparation: Wash the shrimps and leeks, cut the leeks into sections. Fry the shrimps with oil first, add yellow rice wine, soy sauce, vinegar, ginger slices, and other seasonings as desired, and then add the leeks and fry until tender. This dish can treat infertility due to deficiency of the kidneys.

40. Recurrent Miscarriage

Miscarriage is the loss of a fetus before the 20th week of pregnancy or with a fetus weighing less than 1.1 pounds. Recurrent miscarriage refers to three consecutive miscarriages. The main clinical symptoms include vaginal bleeding and paroxysmal abdominal pain. Recurrent miscarriages are always associated with maldevelopment of reproductive organs, immune disorders, endocrine disorders, and various infections of the endometrium.

Pregnant women must develop good living habits and have regular work and rest. It is advisable to ensure eight hours of sleep a night and to do appropriate exercise. Develop the habit of regular defecation and eat more food rich in cellulose to maintain smooth bowel movements. Pregnant women should frequently bathe and change underwear, and especially pay attention to the hygiene of the genitals by cleaning the genital area with warm, clean water every night to prevent infection. Pregnant women should pay attention to adjusting their emotions, try to achieve peace of mind, avoid all kinds of adverse stimuli, eliminate tension, boredom or fear. In particular, they should avoid excessive joyfulness, sadness or anger. These strong emotions can be very unfavorable to fetal growth.

Acupoints of Moxibustion

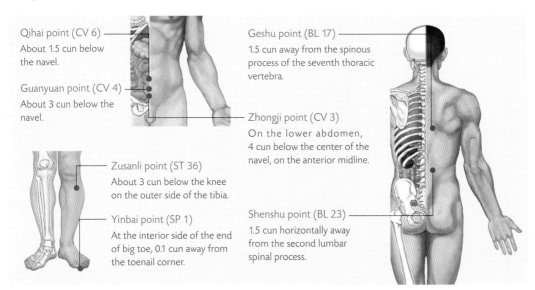

Qihai point (CV 6)
About 1.5 cun below the navel.

Guanyuan point (CV 4)
About 3 cun below the navel.

Geshu point (BL 17)
1.5 cun away from the spinous process of the seventh thoracic vertebra.

Zhongji point (CV 3)
On the lower abdomen, 4 cun below the center of the navel, on the anterior midline.

Zusanli point (ST 36)
About 3 cun below the knee on the outer side of the tibia.

Yinbai point (SP 1)
At the interior side of the end of big toe, 0.1 cun away from the toenail corner.

Shenshu point (BL 23)
1.5 cun horizontally away from the second lumbar spinal process.

Moxibustion Method

Mild moxibustion: Moxibustion is applied to such points as Qihai, Guanyuan, Zhongji, Shenshu, Zusanli, Geshu and Yinbai, beginning with points on the waist and back and then moving to those on the chest and abdomen, working from the upper to lower body. The patient takes an appropriate posture, with the related skin areas exposed. The practitioner ignites a moxa roll at one end and points the ignited end at a point, 3 to 5 centimeters above the skin's surface, until the patient's skin above the point feels warm but with no burning pain. The moxibustion should be given for 15 minutes per point, once a day, for a 10-day course of treatment with an interval of three days between two courses.

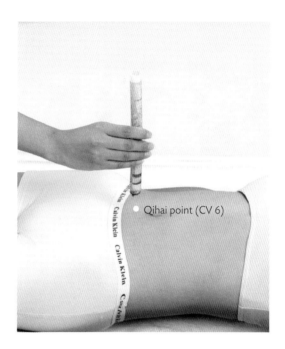

Qihai point (CV 6)

41. Hyperplasia of the Mammary Glands

Hyperplasia of the mammary glands is the most common breast disease in women. It is caused by abnormal mammary gland structure in the breast due to endocrine disorder. Symptoms are characterized by cyclical breast pain, which is aggravated before menstruation each time, but is relieved or disappears after menstruation. In severe cases, pain will be persistent before and after menstruation.

To prevent and cure breast hyperplasia, patients must change their eating habits and lifestyles. Eat less animal fat and tonic, fried and sweet foods. Eat more vegetables and fruits, whole grains, beans, walnuts, black sesame, black fungus, mushrooms and so on. Pay attention to the combination of work and rest and maintain sexual harmony to regulate the endocrine system. Maintain regular routines of daily life and keep the bowel movements smooth. Avoid abuse of contraceptives and operative abortions. Do moderate exercise to strengthen disease resistance .

Acupoints of Moxibustion

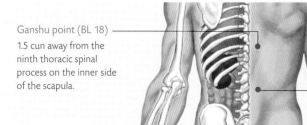

Ganshu point (BL 18)
1.5 cun away from the ninth thoracic spinal process on the inner side of the scapula.

Shenshu point (BL 23)
1.5 cun horizontally away from the second lumbar spinal process.

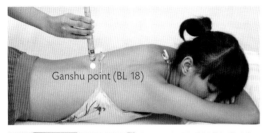
Ganshu point (BL 18)

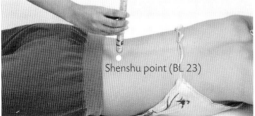
Shenshu point (BL 23)

Moxibustion Method

Mild moxibustion: Moxibustion is applied to the Ganshu and Shenshu points. The patient takes a prone posture. The practitioner ignites a moxa roll at one end and points the ignited end at a point, 3 to 5 centimeters above the skin's surface, until the patient feels warmth without any pain. Moxibustion should be performed 15 to 20 minutes per point, until the skin turns slightly red. This moxibustion should be given once or twice a day for 10 times as a course of treatment, with an interval of 3 to 5 days between two courses.

42. Acute Mastitis

Acute mastitis is an acute inflammation of the breast caused by bacterial infection. It often develops abscesses, and is mostly caused by invasion of lymphatic vessels by staphylococcus aureus or streptococcus. It is most common in breastfeeding women 2 to 6 weeks after giving birth, especially in primipara. The disease can occur at any time during lactation and is most commonly seen at the beginning of breastfeeding.

When one feels breast pain, swelling, or even local skin redness, it's important to breastfeed and drain the breast as much as possible. If necessary, use the suction method to empty the breast or ask a doctor's assistance. Some steps can be taken to prevent mastitis from occurring: First, during the lactation period, wash the nipples with warm water. It is not advisable to let the baby sleep with a nipple in his/her mouth. After breast-feeding, use a bra to hold the breast. Diet should be light, easy to digest and without spicy food. A gloomy mood is also related to this disease. Relieve any trouble, eliminate bad emotions and pay attention to mental conditioning.

Acupoints of Moxibustion

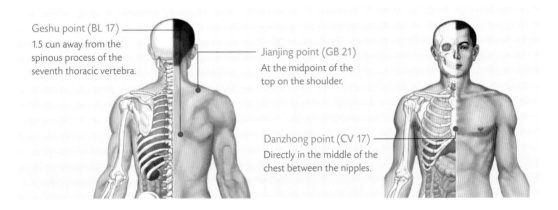

Geshu point (BL 17)
1.5 cun away from the spinous process of the seventh thoracic vertebra.

Jianjing point (GB 21)
At the midpoint of the top on the shoulder.

Danzhong point (CV 17)
Directly in the middle of the chest between the nipples.

Moxibustion Method

Sparrow-pecking moxibustion:
Moxibustion is applied to such points as Jianjing, Danzhong, Geshu and Ashi, moving from points on the waist and back and to those on the chest and abdomen. The patient should take an appropriate posture. The practitioner, standing on one side of the patient, ignites a moxa roll at one end and points the ignited end at the point, 3 to 5 centimeters over the skin's surface. The practitioner holds the roll and moves it up and down, like a sparrow pecking at food. The moxibustion lasts five minutes per point. This is performed once to twice a day,

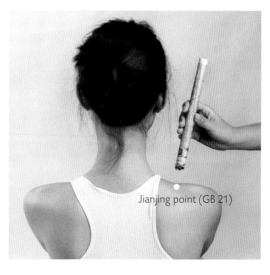
Jianjing point (GB 21)

for 15 times as a course of treatment, with an interval of 3 to 5 days between two courses. During the moxibustion, pay close attention to the temperature of the skin areas under moxibustion to avoid burning the patient's skin.

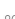

1. Dandelion Porridge
Ingredients: 2.1 ounces of dandelions, 1.1 ounces of honeysuckle, and 1.8 to 3.5 ounces of rice.
    Preparation: Decoct dandelions and honeysuckle, retain the juice after removing the solids, and then add rice to cook a porridge. This porridge can clear heat and expel toxins and is suitable for such symptoms as mastitis, tonsillitis, cholecystitis and conjunctivitis.

2. Daylily Pig's Trotter Soup
Ingredients: 0.5 ounce of fresh daylily roots (or 0.8 ounce of dried daylily), one pig's trotter.
    Preparation: Decoct fresh daylily roots and trotter with water. Eat meat and drink soup once a day, for 3 to 4 consecutive days. The porridge can clear heat, reduce swelling, clear the channels and stimulate milk secretion. It is suitable for mastitis and the lack of milk. Eat this dish on an empty stomach in the morning and evening in autumn and winter.

43. Postpartum Abdominal Pain

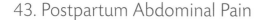

Postpartum abdominal pain refers to the abdominal pain associated with childbirth or childbed occurring in the puerperium. No treatment is needed in mild cases, and the abdominal pain will gradually disappear. Severe or prolonged pain should be treated.

    According to traditional Chinese medicine, the disease is caused by inhibited qi and blood stasis after delivery, excessive postpartum hemorrhage, deficiency of qi and blood, or careless living conditions and a poor mood. Applying moxibustion at related points can promote qi and blood circulation, enhance physical fitness and disperse stagnated liver-qi to relieve depression, thus effectively reducing symptoms.

    Women who have recently had a baby should get out of bed early and gradually increase their physical activities according to their physical strength. Diet should be light, with less raw, cold and flatulence-inducing food. Prevent constipation. Pay attention to keeping the lower abdomen warm to prevent the invasion of pathogenic cold. Stay happy and avoid abdominal pain caused by stagnation of liver-qi.

Acupoints of Moxibustion

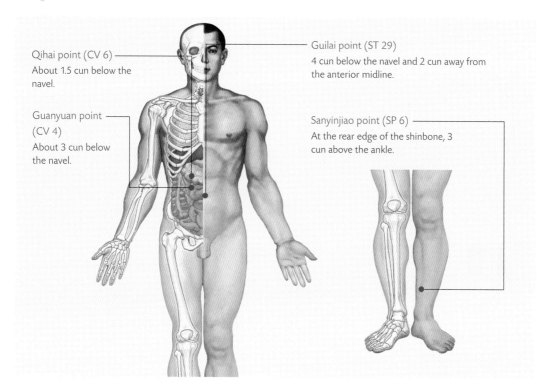

Qihai point (CV 6)
About 1.5 cun below the navel.

Guanyuan point (CV 4)
About 3 cun below the navel.

Guilai point (ST 29)
4 cun below the navel and 2 cun away from the anterior midline.

Sanyinjiao point (SP 6)
At the rear edge of the shinbone, 3 cun above the ankle.

Moxibustion Method

Mild moxibustion: Apply moxibustion to such points as Guanyuan, Guilai, Qihai and Sanyinjiao, beginning with the upper body and moving toward the lower body. The patient should take an appropriate posture. The practitioner ignites a moxa roll at one end and points the ignited end at a point, 3 to 5 centimeters above the skin's surface, until the skin feels warm, without the feeling of burning pain. Apply moxibustion to each acupoint for 15 to 20 minutes, until the skin turns slightly red. Perform one or two times daily for three times as a course of treatment, with an interval of one day between two courses. During moxibustion, the practitioner should be careful to avoid burning the patient's skin with falling ash.

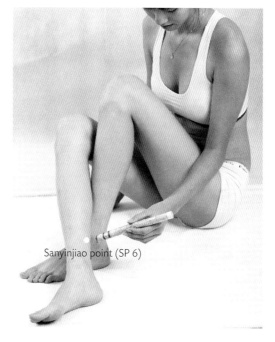

Sanyinjiao point (SP 6)

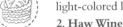

1. Red Bean Pumpkin Powder

Ingredients: 3.5 ounces of red beans, 1.1 ounces of ginger, 7.1 ounces of pumpkin.

   Preparation: Red beans, ginger and pumpkin are baked dry and ground into powder. Administer three times a day, 1.1 ounces each time. This is mainly indicated for postpartum abdominal pain due to blood deficiency, which is manifested by dull and cold pain in the lower abdomen and longing for kneading, a pale complexion, dizziness, tinnitus and small amount of light-colored lochia.

2. Haw Wine

Ingredients: 0.5 ounce of haws, 1.8 ounces of brown sugar, 1.7 ounces of rice wine.

   Preparation: Decoct haws, brown sugar and rice wine with water. Administer three times a day, for seven consecutive days. This is mainly indicated for postpartum abdominal pain due to blood stasis, which is manifested by abdominal pain, refusal to be pressed, lochia with dark purple clots, a pale complexion and a dark tongue.

44. Nausea in Pregnancy

Nausea in pregnancy encompasses several of the main symptoms of gestation, including recurrent nausea, vomiting, anorexia, or vomiting immediately after eating during months two and three of the pregnancy. These symptoms will generally disappear after about 12 weeks pregnancy. They have little effect on work and daily life, and do not require special treatment.

Acupoints of Moxibustion

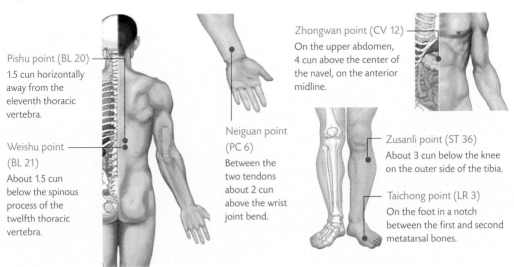

Pishu point (BL 20)
1.5 cun horizontally away from the eleventh thoracic vertebra.

Weishu point (BL 21)
About 1.5 cun below the spinous process of the twelfth thoracic vertebra.

Neiguan point (PC 6)
Between the two tendons about 2 cun above the wrist joint bend.

Zhongwan point (CV 12)
On the upper abdomen, 4 cun above the center of the navel, on the anterior midline.

Zusanli point (ST 36)
About 3 cun below the knee on the outer side of the tibia.

Taichong point (LR 3)
On the foot in a notch between the first and second metatarsal bones.

Moxibustion Method

Mild moxibustion: Moxibustion is applied to such points as Pishu, Weishu, Zhongwan, Neiguan, Zusanli and Taichong, beginning with points on the waist and back and then

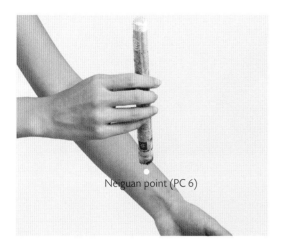
Neiguan point (PC 6)

moving to those on the chest and abdomen, working from the upper to lower body. The patient should take an appropriate posture. The practitioner ignites a moxa roll at one end and points the ignited end at a point, 3 to 5 centimeters above the skin's surface, until the patient's skin feels warm but no burning pain. The moxibustion lasts 10 to 15 minutes for each point, and is given once a day for a five-day course of treatment. If symptoms have not improved, the next course of treatment may be started two days later.

45. Prostatitis

Prostatitis, a common disease in men, refers to the systemic or local symptoms caused by acute or chronic inflammation due to prostate-specific or nonspecific infections. Common symptoms include urgency of urination, frequent urination, burning sensation during urination, or chills, fever, general malaise and other symptoms.

According to traditional Chinese medicine, prostatitis has the closest relationship with the spleen and kidneys. Moxibustion at the relevant points can strengthen the functions of spleen and kidneys and expel damp and heat, thus treating the disease.

Patients with prostatitis should drink plenty of water and urinate frequently. Take medicine with caution because some kinds of medicine will increase the difficulty of urination. Avoid sitting for extended periods. Relax the body and mind and avoid overwork. Maintain a regular sex life. Avoid catching a cold, which can aggravate the illness. Keep the crotch dry and sanitary to reduce the growth of viruses and bacteria. Choose breathable and heat-dissipating cotton underwear.

Acupoints of Moxibustion

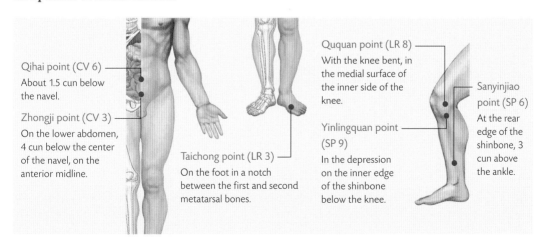

Qihai point (CV 6)
About 1.5 cun below the navel.

Zhongji point (CV 3)
On the lower abdomen, 4 cun below the center of the navel, on the anterior midline.

Taichong point (LR 3)
On the foot in a notch between the first and second metatarsal bones.

Ququan point (LR 8)
With the knee bent, in the medial surface of the inner side of the knee.

Yinlingquan point (SP 9)
In the depression on the inner edge of the shinbone below the knee.

Sanyinjiao point (SP 6)
At the rear edge of the shinbone, 3 cun above the ankle.

Moxibustion Method

Mild moxibustion: Apply moxibustion to such points as Yanglingquan, Sanyinjiao, Qihai, Zhongji, Ququan and Taichong, moving from the upper to lower body. The patient should take an appropriate posture. The practitioner ignites one end of a moxa roll and points the ignited end at a point, 3 to 5 centimeters above the skin's surface, until the patient feels warmth without any pain. Moxibustion lasts 10 to 30 minutes for each point, until the patient's skin turns slightly red. Perform moxibustion once or twice a day for 10 times as a course of treatment, with an interval of 3 to 5 days between two courses.

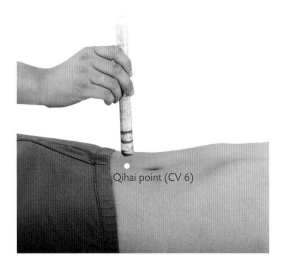

Qihai point (CV 6)

White Gourd Soup with Kelp and Coix Seed
Ingredients: 8.8 ounces of fresh white gourd (with skin), 1.8 ounces of coix seed, 3.5 ounces of kelp.
  Preparation: Wash all ingredients. Cut the white gourd into big pieces and the kelp into thin slices. Put the above ingredients into an earthenware cooking pot and add an appropriate amount of clear water to cook the soup. It serves to clear heat, reduce toxin, facilitate urination and eliminate swelling.

46. Spermatorrhea

Spermatorrhea is a physiological phenomenon of involuntary ejaculation without sexual intercourse. Spermatorrhea while dreaming during sleep is called nocturnal emission, and spermatorrhea without dreaming is called involuntary emission. The frequency of spermatorrhea can range from once every one or two weeks to four or five weeks, which is normal. Spermatorrhea of several times in a week or several times at a night belongs to a pathological phenomenon and should be treated promptly.

Patients with spermatorrhea should not be too nervous, and should aim for psychological regulation to increase confidence in treating the disease. Avoid catching a cold after spermatorrhea, and do not wash with cold water, so as not to be invaded by pathogenic cold. Keep a proper balance between work and rest, do not stay up late, and do not eat spicy or irritating food. Eliminate distracting thoughts and watch fewer pornographic images or movies. Take part in an appropriate amount of athletic activities to divert attention and cultivate sentiments.

Acupoints of Moxibustion

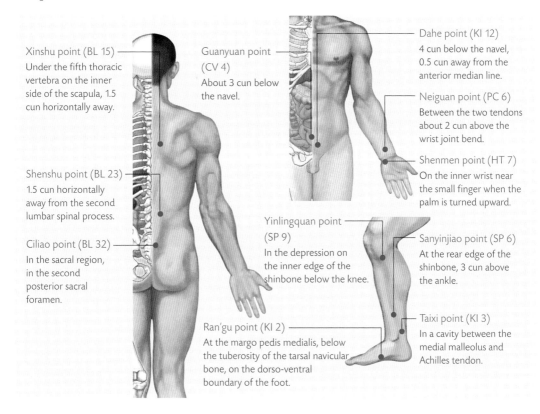

Xinshu point (BL 15)
Under the fifth thoracic vertebra on the inner side of the scapula, 1.5 cun horizontally away.

Guanyuan point (CV 4)
About 3 cun below the navel.

Dahe point (KI 12)
4 cun below the navel, 0.5 cun away from the anterior median line.

Neiguan point (PC 6)
Between the two tendons about 2 cun above the wrist joint bend.

Shenmen point (HT 7)
On the inner wrist near the small finger when the palm is turned upward.

Shenshu point (BL 23)
1.5 cun horizontally away from the second lumbar spinal process.

Ciliao point (BL 32)
In the sacral region, in the second posterior sacral foramen.

Yinlingquan point (SP 9)
In the depression on the inner edge of the shinbone below the knee.

Sanyinjiao point (SP 6)
At the rear edge of the shinbone, 3 cun above the ankle.

Taixi point (KI 3)
In a cavity between the medial malleolus and Achilles tendon.

Ran'gu point (KI 2)
At the margo pedis medialis, below the tuberosity of the tarsal navicular bone, on the dorso-ventral boundary of the foot.

Moxibustion Method

Mild moxibustion: Moxibustion is applied to such points as Xinshu, Shenshu, Ciliao, Guanyuan, Dahe, Neiguan, Shenmen, Yinlingquan, Sanyinjiao, Taixi and Ran'gu, beginning with the points on the waist and back and moving to those on the chest and abdomen, working from the upper to lower body. The patient should take an appropriate position. The practitioner ignites one end of a moxa roll and points the ignited end at a point, 3 to 5 centimeters above the skin's surface. Apply moxibustion to each point for 10 to 20 minutes, until the skin turns slightly red. Perform once daily and repeat 10 days for a course of treatment with an interval of 3 to 5 days between two courses.

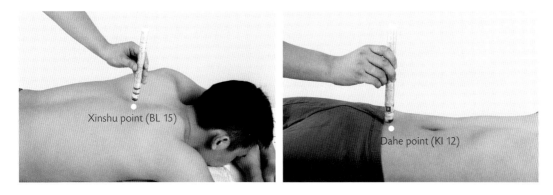

Xinshu point (BL 15)

Dahe point (KI 12)

Stewed Pork Soup with Lotus Seeds and Dried Lilies
Ingredients: 1.1 ounces of lotus seeds, 1.1 ounces of dried lilies, 7.1 to 8.8 ounces of lean pork.
Preparation: Put the lotus seeds, dried lilies and lean pork into a pot, add an appropriate amount of water, and stew it over low heat. Season before eating. This recipe is effective to keep the heart-yang and the kidney-yin in balance and to reinforce the vital essence.

47. Impotence

Impotence is a male condition characterized by the inability to engage in sexual intercourse due to the failure to achieve or maintain an erection, or inability to keep sufficient time of sexual intercourse despite erection and a certain extent of hardness.

According to traditional Chinese medicine, this disease is mainly caused by excessive worry, downward flow of damp-heat, imbalance between heart-yang and kidney-yin, deficiency of qi and blood, and damage to the heart and spleen. Moxibustion at relevant points can nourish the kidneys, regulate qi and blood, expel damp-heat, and replenish the heart and spleen, thereby improving the symptoms.

Moxibustion Methods

Mild moxibustion: Moxibustion is applied to such points as Xinshu, Shenshu, Mingmen, Yaoyangguan, Shenque, Guanyuan, Zhongji, Sanyinjiao and Taixi, working first on points on the waist and back and then those on the chest and abdomen, moving from the upper to lower body. The practitioner ignites a moxa roll at one end and points the ignited end at a point, 3 to 5 centimeters above the skin's surface, until the patient feels warmth but no pain. Apply

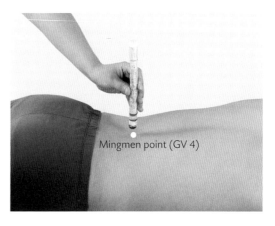
Mingmen point (GV 4)

moxibustion to each point for 15 to 20 minutes. Perform once daily or every two days for a 10-day course of treatment with an interval of 3 to 5 days between two course. This therapy is the most suitable for the impotence caused by debilitation of kidney-yang, the symptoms of which are atrophy or lifted but not firm penis before sexual intercourse, cool semen or ejaculation disorder, accompanied by dizziness, soreness of waist, tinnitus, intolerance to the cold and cold limbs, low spirits, and dark complexion and eye sockets.

Mild moxibustion: Moxibustion is applied to such points as Pangguangshu, Guanyuan, Ququan, Yinlingquan, Sanyinjiao and Ran'gu, beginning with points on the waist and back and moving toward those on the chest and abdomen, working from the upper to lower body. The practitioner ignites a moxa roll at one end and points the ignited end at a point, 3 to 5 centimeters above the skin's surface, until the patient feels warm, without any

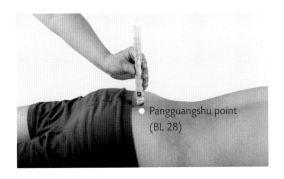

Pangguangshu point
(BL 28)

pain. The moxibustion lasts 10 to 15 minutes for each point. Perform treatment once a day and repeat 10 days for a course of treatment with an interval of 3 to 5 days between two course. This therapy is the most suitable for impotence caused by downward flow of damp-heat, the symptoms of which are weak penis, damp scrotum, fragile waist and knees, and foul yellow urine.

Acupoints of Moxibustion

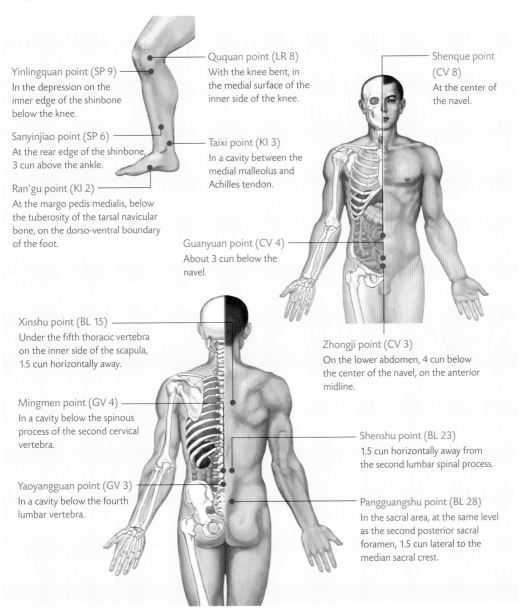

Yinlingquan point (SP 9)
In the depression on the inner edge of the shinbone below the knee.

Ququan point (LR 8)
With the knee bent, in the medial surface of the inner side of the knee.

Shenque point (CV 8)
At the center of the navel.

Sanyinjiao point (SP 6)
At the rear edge of the shinbone, 3 cun above the ankle.

Taixi point (KI 3)
In a cavity between the medial malleolus and Achilles tendon.

Ran'gu point (KI 2)
At the margo pedis medialis, below the tuberosity of the tarsal navicular bone, on the dorso-ventral boundary of the foot.

Guanyuan point (CV 4)
About 3 cun below the navel.

Xinshu point (BL 15)
Under the fifth thoracic vertebra on the inner side of the scapula, 1.5 cun horizontally away.

Zhongji point (CV 3)
On the lower abdomen, 4 cun below the center of the navel, on the anterior midline.

Mingmen point (GV 4)
In a cavity below the spinous process of the second cervical vertebra.

Shenshu point (BL 23)
1.5 cun horizontally away from the second lumbar spinal process.

Yaoyangguan point (GV 3)
In a cavity below the fourth lumbar vertebra.

Pangguangshu point (BL 28)
In the sacral area, at the same level as the second posterior sacral foramen, 1.5 cun lateral to the median sacral crest.

48. Premature Ejaculation

Premature ejaculation is a sexual disorder manifested by ejaculation before the penis enters the vagina, or early ejaculation soon after the penis enters the vagina and before the woman has reached orgasm. Premature ejaculation is mainly marked by physical and psychological causes, which should be promptly treated.

Patients with premature ejaculation can usually take medicine or eat food that can warm yang and invigorate kidneys, such as mutton, river shrimp, young rooster, lobster, shrimp meat, walnut meat, leeks and wolfberry fruit. Eat less spicy and irritating food or raw and cold food, and drink less alcohol, strong tea and coffee. Pay attention to exercise and do more aerobic exercise, as physical health is the key to the treatment of this illness. Patients should try to relieve psychological pressure and should keep a positive attitude about the treatment.

Acupoints of Moxibustion

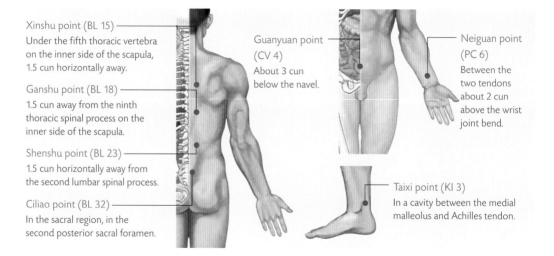

Xinshu point (BL 15)
Under the fifth thoracic vertebra on the inner side of the scapula, 1.5 cun horizontally away.

Ganshu point (BL 18)
1.5 cun away from the ninth thoracic spinal process on the inner side of the scapula.

Shenshu point (BL 23)
1.5 cun horizontally away from the second lumbar spinal process.

Ciliao point (BL 32)
In the sacral region, in the second posterior sacral foramen.

Guanyuan point (CV 4)
About 3 cun below the navel.

Neiguan point (PC 6)
Between the two tendons about 2 cun above the wrist joint bend.

Taixi point (KI 3)
In a cavity between the medial malleolus and Achilles tendon.

Moxibustion Method

Mild moxibustion: Moxibustion is applied to such points as Xinshu, Ganshu, Shenshu, Ciliao, Guanyuan, Neiguan and Taixi, working first with points on the waist and back and then those on the chest and abdomen, moving from the upper to lower body. The patient takes an appropriate posture, with the related skin areas exposed. The practitioner ignites a moxa roll at one end and points the ignited end at a point, 3 to 5 centimeters above the skin's surface, until the patient feels warm, without the feeling of pain. Apply moxibustion to each point for 15 to 20 minutes, until the skin turns slightly red. Perform it once or twice daily for 10 times as a course of treatment, with an interval of 3 to 5 days between two courses. During moxibustion, the practitioner should be careful to keep falling ash from burning the skin.

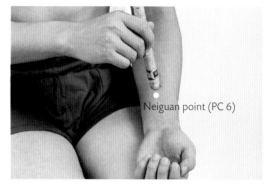

Neiguan point (PC 6)

49. Male Infertility

Male infertility refers to a condition in which the husband and wife have been living together without using contraception for more than two years and the woman is not pregnant, and the woman is examined as normal, but the man is abnormal. There are many causes of male infertility. Impaired sperm production, insufficient sperm amount, poor sperm quality and low sperm motility will all cause male infertility.

Before seeking medical treatment for infertility, men must find out the cause of the illness and treat it symptomatically. Those suffering from infertility should not have excessive psychological pressure and should actively cooperate with the treatment and keep a positive outlook. Patients should get rid of unhealthy habits, avoid staying up late and eat more nutritious food. Quit smoking and drinking, eat less spicy and irritating food, and increase exercise to strengthen the physique. Both husband and wife should work closely together to fight this condition.

Acupoints of Moxibustion

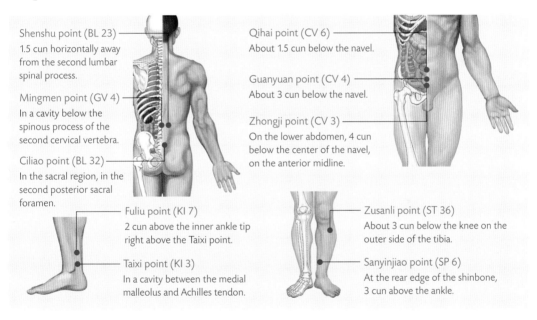

Shenshu point (BL 23)
1.5 cun horizontally away from the second lumbar spinal process.

Mingmen point (GV 4)
In a cavity below the spinous process of the second cervical vertebra.

Ciliao point (BL 32)
In the sacral region, in the second posterior sacral foramen.

Fuliu point (KI 7)
2 cun above the inner ankle tip right above the Taixi point.

Taixi point (KI 3)
In a cavity between the medial malleolus and Achilles tendon.

Qihai point (CV 6)
About 1.5 cun below the navel.

Guanyuan point (CV 4)
About 3 cun below the navel.

Zhongji point (CV 3)
On the lower abdomen, 4 cun below the center of the navel, on the anterior midline.

Zusanli point (ST 36)
About 3 cun below the knee on the outer side of the tibia.

Sanyinjiao point (SP 6)
At the rear edge of the shinbone, 3 cun above the ankle.

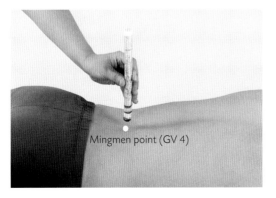

Mingmen point (GV 4)

Moxibustion Method

Mild moxibustion: Moxibustion is applied to Shenshu, Mingmen, Ciliao, Qihai, Guanyuan, Zhongji, Zusanli, Sanyijiao, Fuliu and Taixi points, beginning with points on the waist and back and moving toward those on the chest and abdomen, working from the upper to lower body. The patient should take an appropriate posture. Ignite one end of a moxa roll and point the ignited end at a point, 3 to 5 centimeters above the skin's surface, until the patient feels warmth but no pain. The moxibustion to each point lasts 10 to 30 minutes, once or twice a day for a 30-day course of treatment with an interval of 3 to 5 days between two courses.

1. Coix Seed Porridge

Ingredients: Coix seeds.

　　Preparation: Wash the coix seeds, add water to cook porridge. Eat 8.5 ounces per day on an empty stomach. This has the effect of strengthening the spleen functions, eliminating dampness, clearing the lungs and excreting pus.

2. Black and White Fungus Soup

Ingredients: Black fungus, white fungus, rock candy.

　　Preparation: Use any ratio of black to white fungus. First boil black fungus, and simmer on low heat for three hours. Add white fungus and after boiling, simmer for one hour until it becomes thick. Add an appropriate amount of rock candy. Eat 8.5 ounces daily on an empty stomach. You can also add an appropriate number of Chinese dates in winter. White fungus serves to nourish yin, replenish kidneys, moisten lungs and promote the secretion of body fluid. Black fungus serves to replenish kidneys. The application of both white and black fungus produces the best effect.

50. Obesity

Obesity refers to a certain degree of body weight and overly thick fat layers, causing a state of excessive body fat accumulation. Obesity is a health killer, causing coronary heart disease, diabetes and other diseases. In addition to genetic factors, obesity is also related to the intake of high-fat, high-protein and high-sugar food.

　　Obese patients can achieve weight loss by balancing their diets. Food should be diversified, and patients should eat more vegetables, fruits and potatoes, eat beans and bean products often and eat less fat and animal oil. They should not eat and drink excessively and should maintain an exercise regimen.

Moxibustion Method

Mild moxibustion: Apply moxibustion to such points as Tianshu, Shangjuxu, Sanyinjiao, Quchi, Zusanli, Pishu, Yinlingquan, Fenglong, Zhongwan and Guanyuan, beginning with the points on the waist and back and then moving to those on the chest and abdomen, working from the upper to lower body. The patient should take an appropriate posture. The practitioner ignites one end of a moxa roll and points the ignited end at a point, 3 to 5 centimeters

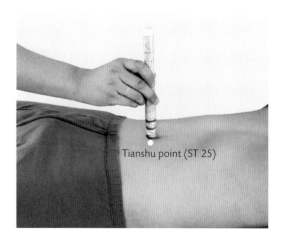
Tianshu point (ST 25)

above the skin's surface, until the patient feels warmth, without any pain. Moxibustion lasts 25 to 30 minutes for each point, until the skin turns slightly red. The moxibustion should be given once daily for a one-month course of treatment with a five-day interval between two courses.

Acupoints of Moxibustion

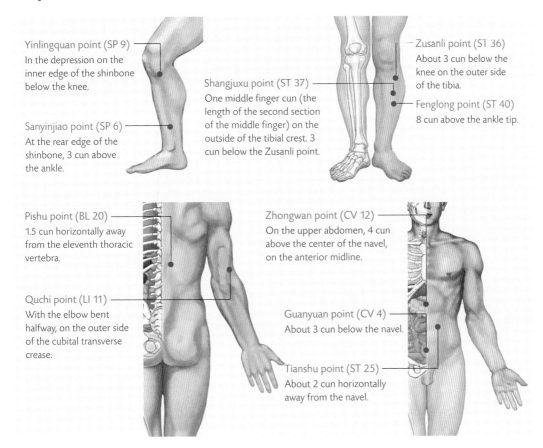

Yinlingquan point (SP 9)
In the depression on the inner edge of the shinbone below the knee.

Sanyinjiao point (SP 6)
At the rear edge of the shinbone, 3 cun above the ankle.

Shangjuxu point (ST 37)
One middle finger cun (the length of the second section of the middle finger) on the outside of the tibial crest. 3 cun below the Zusanli point.

Zusanli point (ST 36)
About 3 cun below the knee on the outer side of the tibia.

Fenglong point (ST 40)
8 cun above the ankle tip.

Pishu point (BL 20)
1.5 cun horizontally away from the eleventh thoracic vertebra.

Quchi point (LI 11)
With the elbow bent halfway, on the outer side of the cubital transverse crease.

Zhongwan point (CV 12)
On the upper abdomen, 4 cun above the center of the navel, on the anterior midline.

Guanyuan point (CV 4)
About 3 cun below the navel.

Tianshu point (ST 25)
About 2 cun horizontally away from the navel.

51. Wrinkles

Wrinkles refer to small lines formed after collagen and active substances in the normal cell membrane tissue are damaged by free radicals, which are developed from the skin tissues under the influence of the external environment. The main reasons for wrinkles are aging, insufficient moisture in the body, or frequent moodiness, impatience, isolation, long-term inadequate sleep and improper use of cosmetics.

Moxibustion Method

Mild moxibustion: Apply moxibustion to such points as Baihui, Yangbai, Yintang, Quanliao, Xiaguan, Yifeng, Futu, Geshu, Shenshu and Shenque, plus Ganshu, Pishu, and Pangguangshu in case of puffiness; and Weishu, Xiaochangshu and Dachangshu for thin and weak patients.

The moxibustion is performed beginning with points on the head and then moving to those on the limbs, working from points on the waist and back and to those on the chest and abdomen, and moving from the upper to lower body. The patient should take an appropriate position. The practitioner ignites one end of a moxa roll and points the ignited end at a point, 3 to 5 centimeters above the skin. Apply moxibustion to each point for 10 minutes. Perform the treatment once a day or once every other day for a 30-day course of treatment with an interval of 3 to 5 days between two courses. When applying moxibustion to the points on the head, the hair should be parted to one side to strengthen the moxibustion's effect.

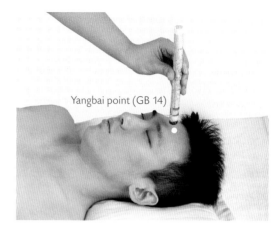

Yangbai point (GB 14)

Acupoints of Moxibustion

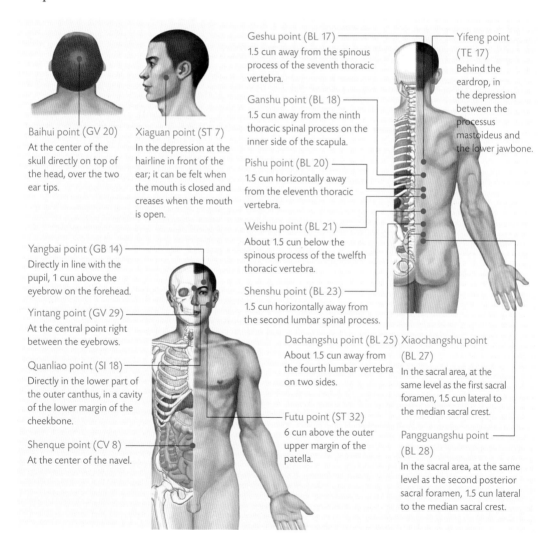

Baihui point (GV 20)
At the center of the skull directly on top of the head, over the two ear tips.

Xiaguan point (ST 7)
In the depression at the hairline in front of the ear; it can be felt when the mouth is closed and creases when the mouth is open.

Yangbai point (GB 14)
Directly in line with the pupil, 1 cun above the eyebrow on the forehead.

Yintang point (GV 29)
At the central point right between the eyebrows.

Quanliao point (SI 18)
Directly in the lower part of the outer canthus, in a cavity of the lower margin of the cheekbone.

Shenque point (CV 8)
At the center of the navel.

Geshu point (BL 17)
1.5 cun away from the spinous process of the seventh thoracic vertebra.

Ganshu point (BL 18)
1.5 cun away from the ninth thoracic spinal process on the inner side of the scapula.

Pishu point (BL 20)
1.5 cun horizontally away from the eleventh thoracic vertebra.

Weishu point (BL 21)
About 1.5 cun below the spinous process of the twelfth thoracic vertebra.

Shenshu point (BL 23)
1.5 cun horizontally away from the second lumbar spinal process.

Dachangshu point (BL 25)
About 1.5 cun away from the fourth lumbar vertebra on two sides.

Futu point (ST 32)
6 cun above the outer upper margin of the patella.

Yifeng point (TE 17)
Behind the eardrop, in the depression between the processus mastoideus and the lower jawbone.

Xiaochangshu point (BL 27)
In the sacral area, at the same level as the first sacral foramen, 1.5 cun lateral to the median sacral crest.

Pangguangshu point (BL 28)
In the sacral area, at the same level as the second posterior sacral foramen, 1.5 cun lateral to the median sacral crest.

52. Chloasma

Chloasma is a pigmentation spot that occurs on the face. It is mainly caused by female endocrine disorder, heavy stress, various diseases (liver and kidney insufficiency, gynecological diseases, diabetes), lack of vitamins and irritation from external chemical drugs.

To eliminate chloasma from the source, first adjust the endocrine system. Have a healthful diet, eat more nutritious vegetables and fruits, mainly high-protein and low-fat food, and drink plenty of water. Ensure adequate sleep, prevent sun exposure and use cosmetics with caution. Exercise more to enhance the physical immunity. Adjust emotions to keep a good mood, which can effectively reduce the occurrence of chloasma.

Acupoints of Moxibustion

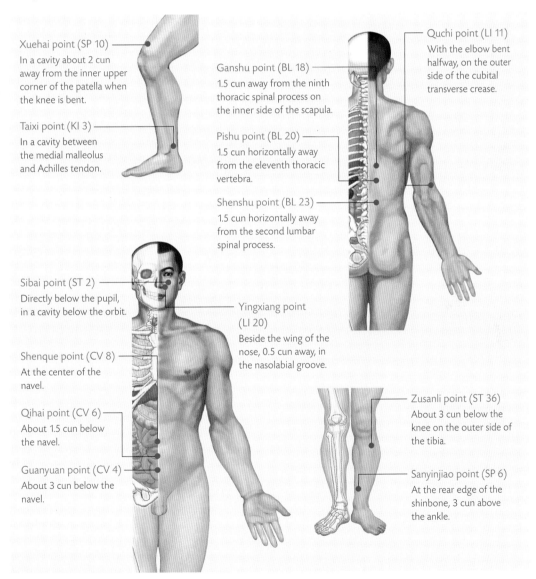

Xuehai point (SP 10)
In a cavity about 2 cun away from the inner upper corner of the patella when the knee is bent.

Taixi point (KI 3)
In a cavity between the medial malleolus and Achilles tendon.

Ganshu point (BL 18)
1.5 cun away from the ninth thoracic spinal process on the inner side of the scapula.

Pishu point (BL 20)
1.5 cun horizontally away from the eleventh thoracic vertebra.

Shenshu point (BL 23)
1.5 cun horizontally away from the second lumbar spinal process.

Quchi point (LI 11)
With the elbow bent halfway, on the outer side of the cubital transverse crease.

Sibai point (ST 2)
Directly below the pupil, in a cavity below the orbit.

Shenque point (CV 8)
At the center of the navel.

Qihai point (CV 6)
About 1.5 cun below the navel.

Guanyuan point (CV 4)
About 3 cun below the navel.

Yingxiang point (LI 20)
Beside the wing of the nose, 0.5 cun away, in the nasolabial groove.

Zusanli point (ST 36)
About 3 cun below the knee on the outer side of the tibia.

Sanyinjiao point (SP 6)
At the rear edge of the shinbone, 3 cun above the ankle.

Moxibustion Methods

Sparrow-pecking moxibustion: Apply moxibustion to such points as Sibai, Yingxiang, Ganshu, Pishu, Shenshu, Qihai, Zusanli, Sanyinjiao and Taixi, and local chloasma areas. Perform moxibustion first on points on the head and face and then those on the limbs, first on points on the waist and back and then those on the chest and abdomen, and working from the upper to lower body. The patient takes an appropriate position. The practitioner ignites one end of a moxa roll and points the ignited end at

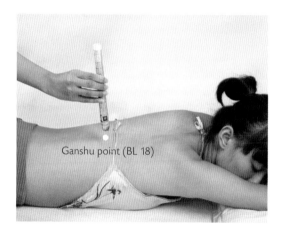

Ganshu point (BL 18)

a point, 3 to 5 centimeters above the skin's surface, and moves the moxa roll up and down, like a sparrow pecking at food. Apply moxibustion to each point for 5 to 10 minutes once every other day for a seven-day course of treatment with an interval of five days between two courses. This therapy is indicated for chloasma due to liver depression, the main symptoms of which are chest and epigastric fullness and distress, pain in both sides of the ribs, vexation and irritability, abdominal distension and loose stool, and irregular menstruation.

Mild moxibustion: Apply moxibustion to such points as Quchi, Xuehai, Sanyinjiao, Ganshu, Pishu, Shenshu, Shenque and Guanyuan, first treating points on the waist and back and then those on the chest and abdomen, moving from upper to lower body. The patient should take an appropriate posture. The practitioner ignites one end of a moxa roll and points the ignited end to a point, 3 to 5 centimeters above the skin's surface, until the patient feels warmth, without the feeling of pain. Moxibustion lasts 15 to 20 minutes for each point, until the skin turns slightly red. This should be performed once a day or once every other day, repeated seven times for a course of treatment with an interval of 3 to 5 days between two courses. This therapy is indicated for chloasma caused by deficiency of spleen and kidneys. The symptoms of deficiency of spleen are sallow complexion, shortness of breath, fatigue, abdominal distension, anorexia and poor menstruation. The symptoms of deficiency of kidneys are dark complexion, dizziness, tinnitus, soreness and weakness of waist and knees and dysphoria in chest, palms and soles.

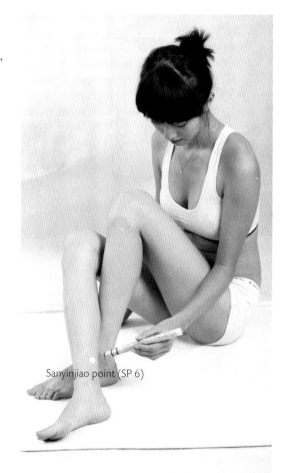

Sanyinjiao point (SP 6)

Green Bean and Lily Skin Whitening Soup

Ingredients: Green beans, red beans, lilies.

Preparation: Wash green beans, red beans and lilies, soak them for half an hour with a proper amount of water. After bringing the mixture to a full boil, lower the heat and simmer until the beans are soft and cooked. Add salt or sugar for seasoning according to personal preference. The vitamins contained in green beans and lilies can reduce melanin and produce a bleaching effect.

53. Freckles

Freckles are light brown spots, with the size ranging from a needle-point to a grain. They are often found on the forehead, bridges of the nose and cheeks, and occasionally on the neck, shoulders and back of the hands.

To reduce or prevent freckles, one must try to avoid prolonged exposure to the sunlight. It is best to wear a hat and use umbrellas and sunscreens when going out. Correct unhealthy habits and ensure adequate rest and sleep. Do not stay up late, smoke or drink liquor. Drink plenty of water, eat more vegetables and fruits, and avoid irritating drinks such as coffee, tea and cola. Keep a good mood.

Acupoints of Moxibustion

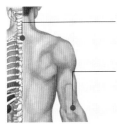

Dazhui point (GV 14)
Under the spinous process of the seventh cervical vertebrae.

Quchi point (LI 11)
With the elbow bent halfway, on the outer side of the cubital transverse crease.

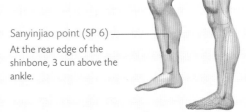

Sanyinjiao point (SP 6)
At the rear edge of the shinbone, 3 cun above the ankle.

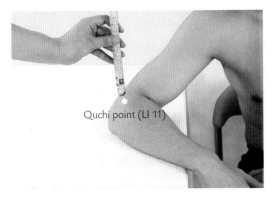

Quchi point (LI 11)

Moxibustion Method

Mild moxibustion: Apply moxibustion to such points as Dazhui, Quchi, Sanyinjiao and local areas with freckles, beginning with points on the head and face and then moving to those on the chest and abdomen. The patient should take an appropriate posture. The practitioner ignites one end of a moxa roll and points the ignited end at a point, 3 to 5 centimeters above the skin's surface, until the patient feels warmth, without the feeling of pain. Moxibustion lasts 10 to 20 minutes for each point, until the skin turns slightly red. Perform therapy once a day or once every other day, repeating 10 times for a course of treatment with an interval of 3 to 5 days between two courses.

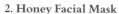

1. Banana Facial Mask

Ingredients: Bananas.

Preparation: Peel bananas and smash them into a paste. Apply paste to the face, and wash away after 15 to 20 minutes. Longtime application can make the facial skin delicate and refreshed. It is especially effective for dry or sensitive skin.

2. Honey Facial Mask

Ingredients: White gourd seeds, peach kernels, honey.

Preparation: Grind the white gourd seeds and peach kernels to a fine powder and add an appropriate amount of honey to mix a thick paste. Apply it to freckles before going to bed every night and wash it away the next morning. After three weeks of application, freckles will gradually become lighter. Pay attention to sun protection during treatment.

54. Rosacea

Rosacea is a chronic skin inflammation that occurs at the center of the face. Cysticercosis, addiction to alcohol and spicy food, hot temperatures, cold stimulation, indigestion and endocrine disorders can all lead to this illness.

To prevent infection, patients must avoid squeezing or scratching the irritated skin and take care to protect the affected area, paying attention to cleaning. Do not use irritating cosmetics. Do not eat spicy and irritating food, keep the bowels open and prevent accumulation of toxins in the body. Reduce sunlight exposure and avoid working in hot and humid environments. Keep regular hours, do not stay up late and avoid overwork to ensure adequate sleep. Strengthen physical exercise to enhance immunity. Stay happy and avoid psychological pressure.

Acupoints of Moxibustion

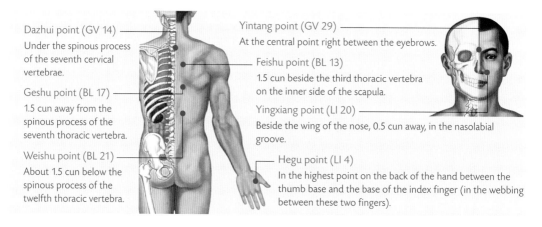

Dazhui point (GV 14)
Under the spinous process of the seventh cervical vertebrae.

Geshu point (BL 17)
1.5 cun away from the spinous process of the seventh thoracic vertebra.

Weishu point (BL 21)
About 1.5 cun below the spinous process of the twelfth thoracic vertebra.

Yintang point (GV 29)
At the central point right between the eyebrows.

Feishu point (BL 13)
1.5 cun beside the third thoracic vertebra on the inner side of the scapula.

Yingxiang point (LI 20)
Beside the wing of the nose, 0.5 cun away, in the nasolabial groove.

Hegu point (LI 4)
In the highest point on the back of the hand between the thumb base and the base of the index finger (in the webbing between these two fingers).

Moxibustion Method

Mild moxibustion: Moxibustion is applied to the Dazhui, Feishu, Geshu, Weishu, Yintang, Yingxiang and Hegu points, working first on points on the head and face and then those on the limbs. The patient should take an appropriate posture. The practitioner ignites one

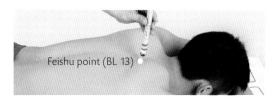
Feishu point (BL 13)

end of a moxa roll and points the ignited end at a point, 3 to 5 centimeters above the skin's surface, until the patient feels warm locally, without the feeling of pain. Apply moxibustion to each point for 15 to 20 minutes, until the patient's local skin turns slightly red. Perform the treatment once to twice a day for 15 times as a course of treatment, with an interval of 3 to 5 days between two courses.

55. Alopecia Areata

Alopecia areata is a sudden onset of local patchy hair disease. The scalp is normal, without inflammation or subjective symptoms. The course of the disease is slow and can resolve and recur spontaneously. It may be related to the dysfunction of the central nervous system and autoimmune diseases.

According to traditional Chinese medicine, this illness is caused by deficiency of kidney-qi, deficiency of qi and blood, deficiency of lung-qi, and blood stasis in the meridians. Moxibustion at relevant points can regulate qi and blood, dredge meridians, and adjust the function of inner organs, thereby improving the symptoms.

Acupoints of Moxibustion

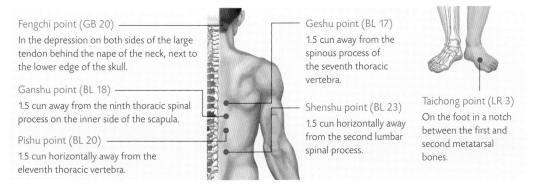

Fengchi point (GB 20)
In the depression on both sides of the large tendon behind the nape of the neck, next to the lower edge of the skull.

Ganshu point (BL 18)
1.5 cun away from the ninth thoracic spinal process on the inner side of the scapula.

Pishu point (BL 20)
1.5 cun horizontally away from the eleventh thoracic vertebra.

Geshu point (BL 17)
1.5 cun away from the spinous process of the seventh thoracic vertebra.

Shenshu point (BL 23)
1.5 cun horizontally away from the second lumbar spinal process.

Taichong point (LR 3)
On the foot in a notch between the first and second metatarsal bones.

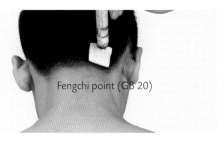
Fengchi point (GB 20)

Moxibustion Method

Mild moxibustion: Moxibustion is applied to the Fengchi, Ganshu, Pishu, Shenshu, Geshu, Taichong points and local areas with alopecia areata, beginning with points on the upper body and then moving to those on the lower body, first treating points on the head and then those on the limbs. The patient should take an appropriate posture. The practitioner ignites one end of a moxa roll and points the ignited end at a point, 3 to 5 centimeters above the skin's surface, until the patient feels warm but has no pain. Apply moxibustion to each point for 5 to 10 minutes, and to the local areas with alopecia areata for 10 to 20 minutes, and repeat once a day for a 10-day course of treatment with an interval of 3 to 5 days between two courses.

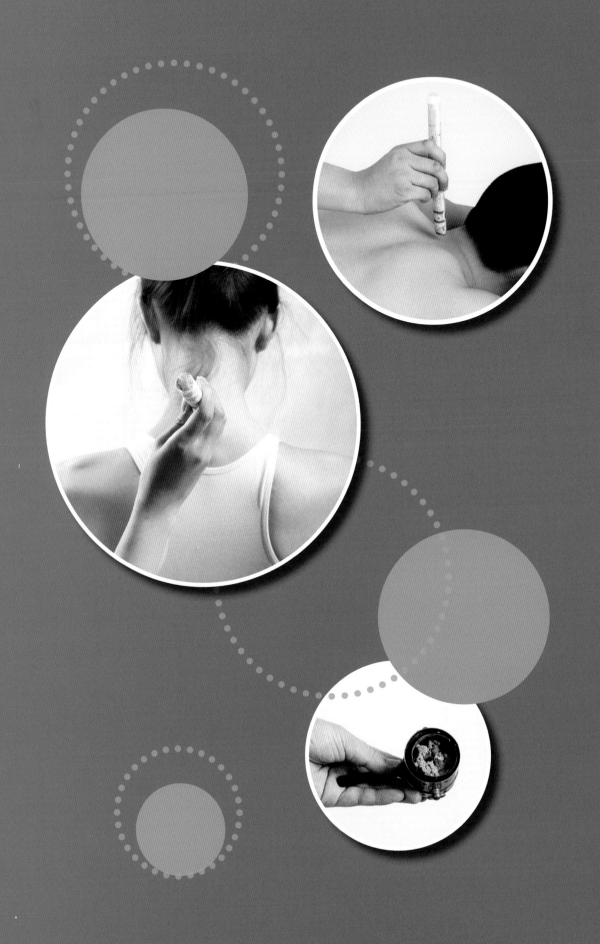

CHAPTER FOUR
Moxibustion Therapy for Chronic Diseases

As people reach middle and old age, the immune system declines and various diseases can occur, including diabetes, high blood pressure, etc. Moxibustion is effective for dredging meridians, expelling dampness and cold, regulating yin and yang and consolidating the physical essence. It can be performed at home as it is safe and effective. The use of moxibustion concurrently with medical treatment can speed up recovery.

1. Diabetes

Diabetes is a condition characterized by high blood sugar. The common symptoms include polyuria, polydipsia, polyphagia and emaciation. It is directly related to overconsumption of fatty and sweet food, excessive drinking, long-term mental irritation and overwork.

Moxibustion at related points can revitalize primordial yang, promote a new balance between yin and yang, restore the function of internal organs and help relieve diabetic conditions.

Diabetics should eat less fried food, and less high-fat and high-cholesterol food such as pigskin, chicken skin and duck skin. Patients should avoid excess salt, and they should use cooking methods like steaming and boiling. They should also eat less sweet food, and eat more food rich in plant fibers, such as fruits and vegetables. They should drink plenty of water, more than 68.3 ounces per day, to facilitate the excretion of metabolic poisons in the body. Properly exercise and maintain a good mood, which will have positive effects on the recovery from the disease.

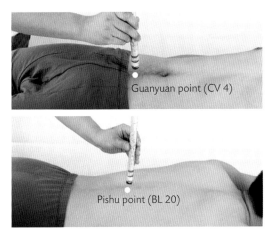

Guanyuan point (CV 4)

Pishu point (BL 20)

Moxibustion Method

Mild moxibustion: Apply moxibustion to such points as Feishu, Pishu, Shenshu, Mingmen, Guanyuan, Zhongwan, Zusanli, Sanyinjiao, Fuliu and Taixi, beginning with points on the back and then moving to those on the chest, and then those on the limbs. The patient can perform moxibustion on points he can reach himself, with the practitioner treating hard-to-reach points. Choose a comfortable position and ignite one end of a moxa roll. Point it at the point, 3 to 5 centimeters from the skin's surface, until the patient feels comfortable but has no burning pain. Moxibustion lasts 5 to 10 minutes for each point, until the local skin turns slightly red. This treatment should be performed once a day for a 10-day course of treatment, with an interval of 3 to 5 days between two courses.

Acupoints of Moxibustion

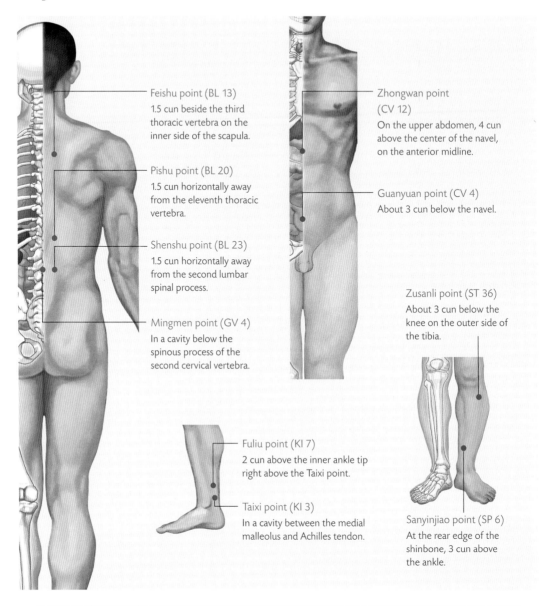

Feishu point (BL 13)
1.5 cun beside the third thoracic vertebra on the inner side of the scapula.

Pishu point (BL 20)
1.5 cun horizontally away from the eleventh thoracic vertebra.

Shenshu point (BL 23)
1.5 cun horizontally away from the second lumbar spinal process.

Mingmen point (GV 4)
In a cavity below the spinous process of the second cervical vertebra.

Zhongwan point (CV 12)
On the upper abdomen, 4 cun above the center of the navel, on the anterior midline.

Guanyuan point (CV 4)
About 3 cun below the navel.

Zusanli point (ST 36)
About 3 cun below the knee on the outer side of the tibia.

Fuliu point (KI 7)
2 cun above the inner ankle tip right above the Taixi point.

Taixi point (KI 3)
In a cavity between the medial malleolus and Achilles tendon.

Sanyinjiao point (SP 6)
At the rear edge of the shinbone, 3 cun above the ankle.

Mushroom with Cabbage

Ingredients: 0.2 ounce of mushrooms, 8.8 ounces of cabbage, 0.4 ounce of soy sauce, 0.1 ounce of salt, 0.4 ounce of vegetable oil, 0.1 of ounce sugar.

Preparation: Remove the mushroom stalks and immerse mushrooms in warm water to wash, retaining the first soaking water. Wash the cabbage and cut into one-inch sections. After the pan is warmed, add the cabbage to the pan. When cabbage is half-cooked, add the mushrooms, soy sauce, salt and sugar, and add the first soaking water. Cover it with a lid and continue to cook until it is tasty. Mushrooms contain lots of plant fiber, which prevents constipation, promotes the expulsion of toxins, reduces cholesterol, and prevents diabetes and large intestine cancer. Moreover, mushrooms are low in calories and conducive to weight management.

2. Hypertension

Hypertension is a systemic chronic disease characterized by an increase in diastolic pressure and/or systolic pressure. It is often accompanied by headache, dizziness, tinnitus and insomnia. It can also lead to heart, brain and kidney lesions.

According to traditional Chinese medicine, the disease is caused by emotional depression, excessive mental stress, excessive drinking and intake of fatty, sweet or strong-flavored food. Moxibustion at the corresponding points can regulate yang in the whole body and improve disease resistance, thus lowering blood pressure.

Hypertensive patients should pay attention to diet, eat less salty and fatty food, and avoid eating high-cholesterol foods such as animal organs. Obese people need to control their diet to lose weight; they should also avoid smoking and alcohol. Patients should pay attention to a proper balance between work and rest, do aerobic exercise, and ensure adequate sleep. Keeping a positive mood is also helpful in lowering blood pressure.

Acupoints of Moxibustion

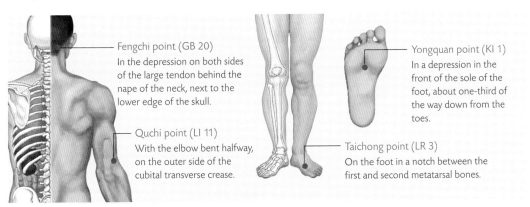

Fengchi point (GB 20)
In the depression on both sides of the large tendon behind the nape of the neck, next to the lower edge of the skull.

Quchi point (LI 11)
With the elbow bent halfway, on the outer side of the cubital transverse crease.

Yongquan point (KI 1)
In a depression in the front of the sole of the foot, about one-third of the way down from the toes.

Taichong point (LR 3)
On the foot in a notch between the first and second metatarsal bones.

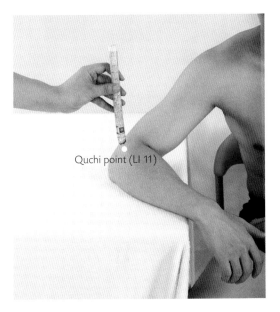

Quchi point (LI 11)

Moxibustion Method

Mild moxibustion: Moxibustion is applied to the Fengchi, Quchi, Taichong and Yongquan points, beginning with points on the head and then moving to those on the limbs. The patient should choose a comfortable posture for each acupoint, rather than trying to maintain any one position for a long time. Ignite a moxa roll at one end and point it at a point, 2 to 3 centimeters from the skin, until the skin feels warm, without a feeling of burning pain. Moxibustion lasts 10 minutes for each point, until the skin reddens. This treatment should be applied once a day for three times as a course of treatment, with an interval of 3 to 5 days between two courses. Place a slice of ginger over Fengchi point to prevent burning the hair with falling ash.

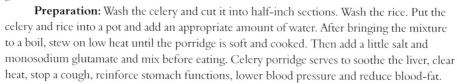

1. Celery Porridge

Ingredients: 4.2 ounces of celery with root, 8.8 ounces of rice, a little salt and monosodium glutamate.

Preparation: Wash the celery and cut it into half-inch sections. Wash the rice. Put the celery and rice into a pot and add an appropriate amount of water. After bringing the mixture to a boil, stew on low heat until the porridge is soft and cooked. Then add a little salt and monosodium glutamate and mix before eating. Celery porridge serves to soothe the liver, clear heat, stop a cough, reinforce stomach functions, lower blood pressure and reduce blood-fat.

2. Peanuts Soaked with Vinegar

Ingredients: Any number of raw peanuts and vinegar.

Preparation: Soak raw peanuts in vinegar and eat them after five days, 10 to 15 peanuts every morning. This food helps reduce blood pressure, stop bleeding and lower cholesterol.

3. Hyperlipidemia

Hyperlipidemia is a common disease among middle-aged and elderly people. Most patients do not have any symptoms or signs; the condition is mostly found during blood biochemical tests. Hyperlipidemia can cause hypertension, atherosclerosis, coronary heart disease and other cardiovascular and cerebrovascular diseases. Patients should pay attention to it.

Hyperlipidemia is mainly related to disorderly diet, emotional disorder, and weak health due to old age. Patients must regulate their diets, strictly controlling the intake of cholesterol and eating more fresh vegetables, fruits, soy products, etc., as well as changing cooking methods by using less oil and using a stewing method for cooking or having cold vegetable dishes in sauce. Set a limit on sweets and avoid alcohol and tobacco. Strengthen and persist in physical activity to help burn fat and enhance physical resistance. Keep a good mood and avoid over-strain to help treat the disease.

Moxibustion Method

Swirling moxibustion: Apply moxibustion to Pishu and Weishu points. The patient should take a prone posture, as the practitioner stands on one side of the patient. Point the ignited moxa roll at a point, about 3 centimeters above the skin's surface, then move it left and right horizontally or circularly, until the skin feels warm, without a feeling of pain. The moxibustion lasts 10 to 15 minutes for each point. Preform the moxibustion once every day, for 10 days as a course of treatment, with an interval of 3 to 5 days between two courses. During moxibustion, the practitioner should be careful to avoid burning the skin with falling ash in the process of movement or rotation.

Acupoints of Moxibustion

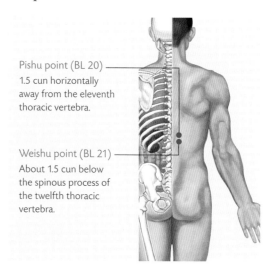

Pishu point (BL 20)
1.5 cun horizontally away from the eleventh thoracic vertebra.

Weishu point (BL 21)
About 1.5 cun below the spinous process of the twelfth thoracic vertebra.

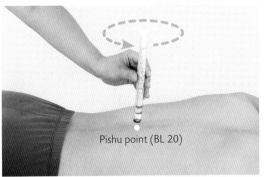

Pishu point (BL 20)

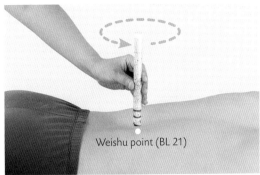

Weishu point (BL 21)

4. Asthma

Asthma is a chronic airway inflammation that can cause recurrent wheezing, shortness of breath, chest tightness and cough, mostly attacking at night or in the early morning.

According to traditional Chinese medicine, the treatment of asthma should focus on mediating lung, spleen, and kidney functions. Moxibustion at the corresponding points can regulate organ function and improve the symptoms.

Patients should have a light diet, avoid spicy and irritating food, and ensure an adequate and balanced variety of nutrients to enhance immunity and prevent respiratory infections. Avoid catching colds because they can cause respiratory infections and trigger asthma. Persist in walking and jogging to improve and enhance lung functions. Keep emotional stability.

Acupoints of Moxibustion

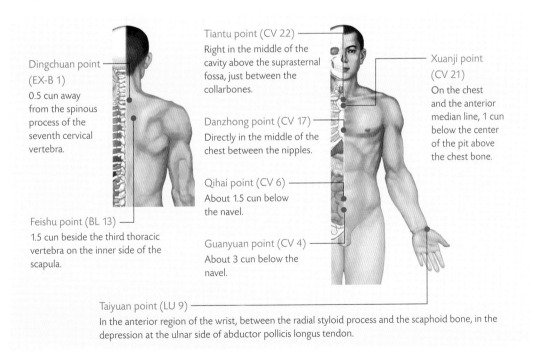

Dingchuan point (EX-B 1)
0.5 cun away from the spinous process of the seventh cervical vertebra.

Feishu point (BL 13)
1.5 cun beside the third thoracic vertebra on the inner side of the scapula.

Tiantu point (CV 22)
Right in the middle of the cavity above the suprasternal fossa, just between the collarbones.

Danzhong point (CV 17)
Directly in the middle of the chest between the nipples.

Qihai point (CV 6)
About 1.5 cun below the navel.

Guanyuan point (CV 4)
About 3 cun below the navel.

Xuanji point (CV 21)
On the chest and the anterior median line, 1 cun below the center of the pit above the chest bone.

Taiyuan point (LU 9)
In the anterior region of the wrist, between the radial styloid process and the scaphoid bone, in the depression at the ulnar side of abductor pollicis longus tendon.

Moxibustion Method

Mild moxibustion: Moxibustion is applied to such points as Dingchuan, Feishu, Tiantu, Xuanji, Danzhong, Qihai, Guanyuan and Taiyuan, beginning with the back, then the chest and abdomen, and then the limbs. The patient should choose a comfortable posture for moxibustion at each acupoint, to avoid maintaining a difficult posture for a long time. The practitioner ignites one end of a moxa roll and points the ignited end at a point, 3 to 5 centimeters above the skin's surface, until the patient feels warmth but no pain. Moxibustion lasts 5 to 10 minutes for each point, until the patient feels comfortable and the targeted skin area reddens. Such treatment should be given once a day or once every other day for a five-day course of treatment, with an interval of 3 to 5 days between two courses.

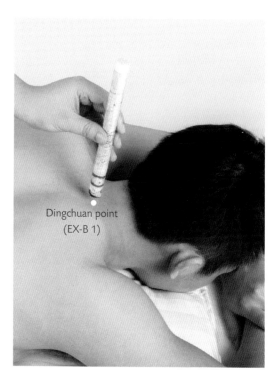

Dingchuan point
(EX-B 1)

1. Ginkgo Syrup

Ingredients: 1.8 ounces of ginkgoes, appropriate amount of sugar.

Preparation: Fry the ginkgoes on low heat, beat the skin open with a knife, remove the shell and coat, wash and cut into small slices. Wash the pot and add water and ginkgoes. Bring to a boil on high heat, then lower the heat and cook for a short time. Add sugar and bring to a boil before serving. Ginkgo in sugar water serves to strengthen lung functions and stop asthma.

2. Almond Porridge

Ingredients: 0.4 ounce of almonds, 1.8 ounces of rice, appropriate amount of rock candy.

Preparation: Peel the almonds and grind them into a fine powder. Decoct it with water, strain and retain the liquid. Then add rice, rock candy and water to cook into a porridge. Take it warm twice a day, helping to clear the lungs, eliminate phlegm and stop coughing and asthma. This is a good medicine for the treatment of cough and asthma.

5. Chronic Bronchitis

Chronic bronchitis is a chronic, nonspecific inflammation of the trachea, bronchial mucosa, and surrounding tissue caused by infectious or noninfective factors. The main symptoms are cough, sputum and asthma that last for more than three months. Smoking, air pollution and allergies can all cause chronic bronchitis.

According to traditional Chinese medicine, the main causes of bronchitis are deficiency of the spleen, lungs and kidneys, as well as excess heat in the liver and lungs. Moxibustion at the corresponding points can improve organ function and regulate the functional activities of qi, thereby improving the symptoms.

Patients with chronic bronchitis should avoid inhaling any dust, powder or irritating gas, as these induce chronic bronchitis. It's important to pay attention to keeping warm in the cold season to avoid catching a cold, and to exercise regularly, as exercise can improve the physical immune system and heart and lung functions. Patients should also quit smoking and drink alcohol in moderation. In terms of diet, food should not be too salty; avoid fried and gas-producing food, and eat high-protein, high-calorie, high-vitamin, low-fat, and easily digestible food such as lean meat, eggs, milk, fish, vegetables and fruits. Maintain a good mood.

Acupoints of Moxibustion

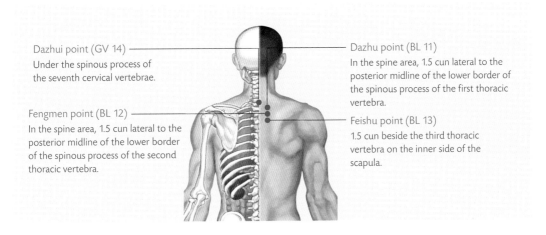

Dazhui point (GV 14)
Under the spinous process of the seventh cervical vertebrae.

Dazhu point (BL 11)
In the spine area, 1.5 cun lateral to the posterior midline of the lower border of the spinous process of the first thoracic vertebra.

Fengmen point (BL 12)
In the spine area, 1.5 cun lateral to the posterior midline of the lower border of the spinous process of the second thoracic vertebra.

Feishu point (BL 13)
1.5 cun beside the third thoracic vertebra on the inner side of the scapula.

Moxibustion Method

Mild moxibustion: Moxibustion is applied to such points as Fengmen, Dazhui, Dazhu and Feishu. The patient takes a prone posture. The practitioner, standing on one side of the patient, ignites one end of a moxa roll and points the ignited end at a point, 3 to 5 centimeters above the skin's surface, until the patient's local skin feels warm, without any pain. Moxibustion lasts 15 to 20 minutes, until the skin reddens. For a patient with decreased sensitivity, the practitioner can place an index finger and a middle finger on both sides of the point to feel the temperature and avoid burning the skin. This moxibustion should be applied once or twice a day for 10 times as a course of treatment, with an interval of 3 to 5 days between two courses.

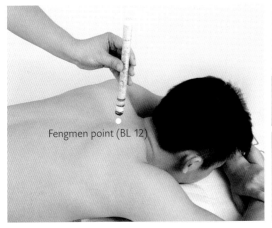

Fengmen point (BL 12)

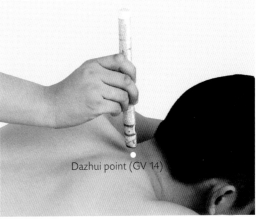

Dazhui point (GV 14)

6. Coronary Heart Disease

Coronary heart disease, short for coronary atherosclerotic heart disease, is a common heart disease. It is manifested as a squeezing pain in the center of the chest and can be transmitted to the neck, lower jaw, arms, back and stomach. Other possible symptoms are dizziness, shortness of breath, sweating, chills, nausea and fainting. Patients with severe cases may die of heart failure.

Patients should develop a healthy and reasonable diet, avoiding excessive fats and sweets, adopting low-salt, low-fat, low-cholesterol and high-fiber dietary principles. Avoid overeating, alcohol and tobacco. Maintain a proper balance between work and rest, avoid heavy physical work, and ensure adequate sleep. Actively participate in physical exercise to enhance heart function and promote metabolism. Patients with coronary heart disease should carry emergency medication with them so they can take medicine promptly at the time of onset.

Moxibustion Methods

Mild moxibustion: Moxibustion is applied to such points as Xinshu, Jueyinshu, Juque, Danzhong and Neiguan, beginning with points on the back and moving to those on the chest and abdomen. The patient takes a comfortable posture. The practitioner, standing on one side of the patient, ignites one end of a moxa roll and points the ignited end at a point, 3 to 5 centimeters above the skin's surface, until the patient's skin feels warmth but no pain. Moxibustion lasts 15 to

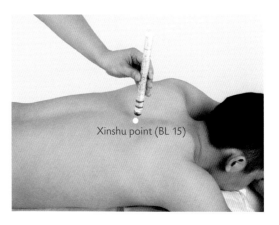

Xinshu point (BL 15)

20 minutes for each point, until the local skin turns slightly red. Perform the therapy once or twice daily for 10 times as a course of treatment, with 3 to 5 days between two courses.

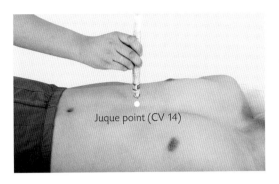

Juque point (CV 14)

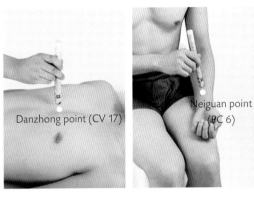

Danzhong point (CV 17)

Neiguan point (PC 6)

Mild moxibustion: Moxibustion is applied to such points as Xinshu, Danzhong, Juque, Tongli, Jianshi, Neiguan, and Zusanli, beginning with points on the back and then moving to those on the chest and abdomen, working from the upper to lower body. The patient takes a comfortable posture. The practitioner ignites one end of a moxa roll and points the ignited end at a point, 3 to 5 centimeters above the skin's surface. The patient should not move during moxibustion, to avoid burning the skin. During the moxibustion, the patient should feel warmth without any feeling of pain. Apply moxibustion to each point for 15 to 20 minutes, until the patient feels comfortable and the local skin turns slightly red. Perform the therapy once a day or once every other day and repeat it 10 times for a course of treatment, with an interval of 3 to 5 days between two courses.

Acupoints of Moxibustion

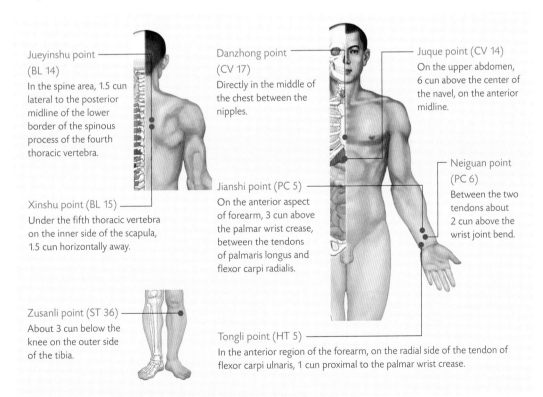

Jueyinshu point (BL 14)
In the spine area, 1.5 cun lateral to the posterior midline of the lower border of the spinous process of the fourth thoracic vertebra.

Danzhong point (CV 17)
Directly in the middle of the chest between the nipples.

Juque point (CV 14)
On the upper abdomen, 6 cun above the center of the navel, on the anterior midline.

Xinshu point (BL 15)
Under the fifth thoracic vertebra on the inner side of the scapula, 1.5 cun horizontally away.

Jianshi point (PC 5)
On the anterior aspect of forearm, 3 cun above the palmar wrist crease, between the tendons of palmaris longus and flexor carpi radialis.

Neiguan point (PC 6)
Between the two tendons about 2 cun above the wrist joint bend.

Zusanli point (ST 36)
About 3 cun below the knee on the outer side of the tibia.

Tongli point (HT 5)
In the anterior region of the forearm, on the radial side of the tendon of flexor carpi ulnaris, 1 cun proximal to the palmar wrist crease.

7. Fatty Liver Disease

Fatty liver disease refers to excessive accumulation of fat in the liver cells. Patients with mild cases are asymptomatic or only feel tired, and most patients with fatty liver disease are relatively overweight, so it is more difficult to find mild subjective symptoms. In moderate and severe cases, there are symptoms similar to those of chronic hepatitis, which may include lack of appetite, fatigue, nausea, vomiting, emaciation and pain in the liver area or upper right abdomen.

Patients with fatty liver disease should develop and maintain a healthy and reasonable diet-plan to control calorie intake, and often eat lean meat, egg white, fishes and fresh vegetables. Limit cholesterol intake and eat less high-cholesterol food such as egg yolk, fish eggs, squid. Do not drink alcohol, as it can greatly damage the liver. Exercise properly to help decrease body fat. Take medicine with caution because the side effects of medicine can damage the liver. Patients are advised to relax their emotions, learn to control their anger and maintain a positive mood.

Acupoints of Moxibustion

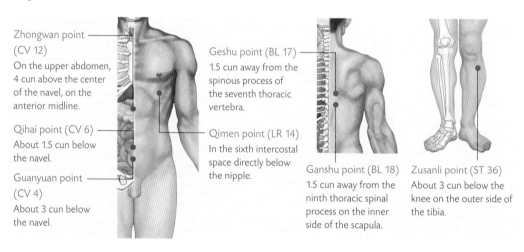

Zhongwan point (CV 12)
On the upper abdomen, 4 cun above the center of the navel, on the anterior midline.

Qihai point (CV 6)
About 1.5 cun below the navel.

Guanyuan point (CV 4)
About 3 cun below the navel.

Qimen point (LR 14)
In the sixth intercostal space directly below the nipple.

Geshu point (BL 17)
1.5 cun away from the spinous process of the seventh thoracic vertebra.

Ganshu point (BL 18)
1.5 cun away from the ninth thoracic spinal process on the inner side of the scapula.

Zusanli point (ST 36)
About 3 cun below the knee on the outer side of the tibia.

Moxibustion Methods

Moxibustion with moxa stick roll holder and mild moxibustion: The patient should take a supine posture. Choose a large-sized moxa stick roll holder, and place it on the Zhongwan, Guanyuan and Qihai points. Ignite a moxa roll and put it on the mesh, and then close the cover to perform moxibustion. Moxibustion lasts 15 to 20 minutes for each point. This therapy is characterized by evenly distributed heat that makes the patient feel comfortable. Next take two moxa rolls, one in each hand, and

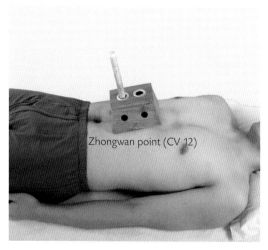

Zhongwan point (CV 12)

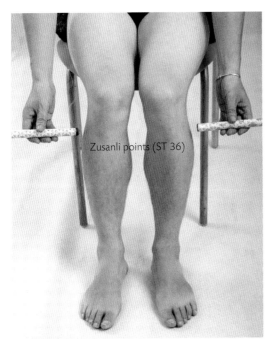

Zusanli points (ST 36)

aim them at the Zusanli points on the two legs respectively. This is performed 3 to 5 centimeters from the skin's surface and lasts 10 minutes, until the skin reddens. Such treatment should be given once or twice a day for 10 times as a course of treatment, with an interval of 3 to 5 days between two courses. This method is applicable to patients with fatty liver disease caused by deficiency of the spleen and stomach. The symptoms include more than normal discharge of excrement if the patients eat oily food or eat a bit more than usual, along with undigested food. The excrement is sometimes watery, recurring for a long time, together with the decline of appetite. Stuffiness felt after the meal, sallow complexion, low spirits, pale tongue surface and weak pulse are also symptoms.

Mild moxibustion: Moxibustion is applied to such points as Geshu, Ganshu, Qimen and Zusanli, beginning with the points on the back and moving to those on the chest and abdomen, working from the upper to lower body. The patient takes an appropriate posture. The practitioner, standing on one side of the patient, ignites a moxa roll at one side and aims it at a point, 3 to 5 centimeters from the skin's surface, until the patient's skin feels warm, without the feeling of pain. Apply moxibustion to each point for 15 to 20 minutes, until local skin turns slightly red. Perform it once or twice a day for 10 times as a course of treatment, with an interval of 3 to 5 days between two courses.

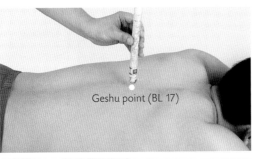

Geshu point (BL 17)

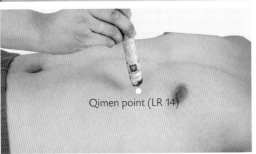

Qimen point (LR 14)

Spinach Egg Soup

Ingredients: 7.1 ounces of spinach, two eggs, appropriate amount of salt and monosodium glutamate.

   Preparation: Wash spinach and fry it in a pot, then add an appropriate amount of water. Bring to a boil and add the eggs, then add salt and monosodium glutamate for seasoning before eating. The soup with spinach and eggs serves to reduce weight and blood-fat, moisten intestines, facilitate bowel movement and relieve fatty liver disease.

8. Cirrhosis

Cirrhosis is a common chronic liver disease of scar tissue formed in response to damage, which can result from one or more causes. The early symptoms of liver cirrhosis are not obvious and can be manifested by fatigue, anorexia, emaciation and facial darkness. In the later stage, there will be splenomegaly, ascites, liver dysfunction and so on.

Patients with cirrhosis should regulate their diets, mainly eating high-protein, high-vitamin, high-calorie and easily digestible food. Do not drink alcohol; drink less tea. Develop normal schedules to ensure adequate sleep and avoid overwork. Learn to control emotions, eliminate worries and anger, and stay calm, which is conducive to physical rehabilitation. Do not take medicine improperly to avoid increasing the burden on the liver. Do appropriate physical exercise such as walking and *taijiquan* (a kind of traditional Chinese martial art), aiming for a suitable amount of exercise without feeling tired.

Acupoints of Moxibustion

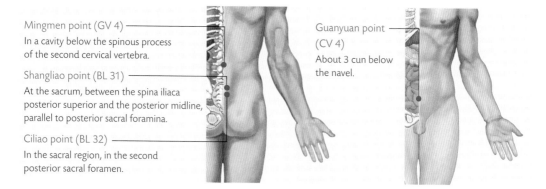

Mingmen point (GV 4)
In a cavity below the spinous process of the second cervical vertebra.

Shangliao point (BL 31)
At the sacrum, between the spina iliaca posterior superior and the posterior midline, parallel to posterior sacral foramina.

Ciliao point (BL 32)
In the sacral region, in the second posterior sacral foramen.

Guanyuan point (CV 4)
About 3 cun below the navel.

Moxibustion Method

Mild moxibustion: Moxibustion is applied to such points as Mingmen, Guanyuan, Shangliao and Ciliao, beginning with points on the back and then moving to points on the chest and abdomen. The patient takes a comfortable posture. The practitioner, standing on one side of the patient and holding a moxa roll, ignites the moxa roll at one end and points the ignited end at a point, 3 to 5 centimeters above the skin's surface, until the patient feels warmth but no pain. Moxibustion lasts 20 to 30 minutes, until the patient feels comfortable and the related skin area reddens. Perform the therapy once

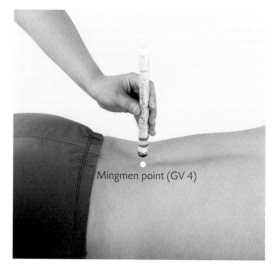

Mingmen point (GV 4)

or twice a day, 10 times for a course of treatment with an interval of 3 to 5 days between two courses. This therapy is the most suitable for the middle stage of cirrhosis.

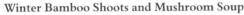

Winter Bamboo Shoots and Mushroom Soup

Ingredients: 8.8 ounces of bamboo shoots and 1.8 ounces of mushrooms.

   Preparation: Wash, peel and slice the winter bamboo shoots, and wash and slice the mushrooms. Put them into a pot and fry for about 10 minutes, then add soup and seasoning and simmer until boil. This recipe is helpful to patients with cirrhosis manifested by fatigue, anorexia, abdominal distension, etc. It has the effect of strengthening the spleen functions and soothing the liver.

9. Palpitations

Palpitations are feelings of a fast-beating or pounding heart. When they occur, the patient feels the heartbeat is fast and strong, or fluttering, accompanied by discomfort in the precordial area. This symptom can be found in many diseases, often coexisting with insomnia, forgetfulness, dizziness and tinnitus.

   Patients with heart palpitations should pay attention to diet regulation, eat nutritious and digestible food, eat less food containing animal fat, and less salty, spicy and irritating food. It's important for patients to participate in physical exercise, such as walking and *taijiquan*, but not to exercise too much, to avoid causing palpitations. Patients should pay attention to adjusting emotions and try to avoid negative emotions such as panic, irritation, worry and exasperation. Keep a calm and happy mood.

Acupoints of Moxibustion

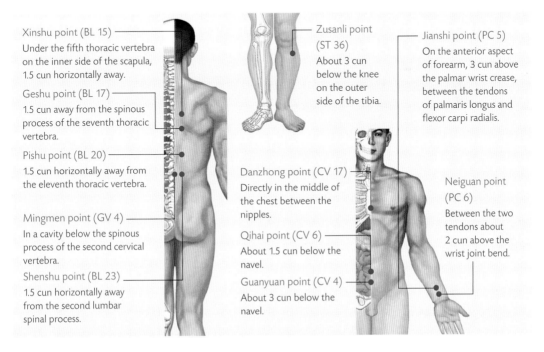

Xinshu point (BL 15)
Under the fifth thoracic vertebra on the inner side of the scapula, 1.5 cun horizontally away.

Geshu point (BL 17)
1.5 cun away from the spinous process of the seventh thoracic vertebra.

Pishu point (BL 20)
1.5 cun horizontally away from the eleventh thoracic vertebra.

Mingmen point (GV 4)
In a cavity below the spinous process of the second cervical vertebra.

Shenshu point (BL 23)
1.5 cun horizontally away from the second lumbar spinal process.

Zusanli point (ST 36)
About 3 cun below the knee on the outer side of the tibia.

Danzhong point (CV 17)
Directly in the middle of the chest between the nipples.

Qihai point (CV 6)
About 1.5 cun below the navel.

Guanyuan point (CV 4)
About 3 cun below the navel.

Jianshi point (PC 5)
On the anterior aspect of forearm, 3 cun above the palmar wrist crease, between the tendons of palmaris longus and flexor carpi radialis.

Neiguan point (PC 6)
Between the two tendons about 2 cun above the wrist joint bend.

Moxibustion Methods

Mild moxibustion: Moxibustion is applied to such points as Xinshu, Pishu, Geshu, Danzhong, Qihai, Guanyuan, Jianshi, Neiguan and Zusanli, beginning with points on the back and then the chest and abdomen, moving from the upper to lower body. The practitioner, standing on one side of the patient, ignites a moxa roll at one side and aims it at a point, 3 to 5 centimeters from the skin's surface, until the patient's skin feels warm, without the feeling of pain. Moxibustion lasts 15 to 20 minutes for each point, until the skin turns slightly red. Such treatment should be given once daily for a 10-day course of treatment with an interval of five days between two courses. It is mainly suitable for patients with deficiency of qi and blood. Qi deficiency is marked by the fear of coldness and cold limbs, sweating, dizziness, tinnitus, low spirits, fatigue, palpitations, difficulty in breathing and developmental delay. Blood deficiency is characterized by sallow complexion, dry skin, withered hair, dry and split nails, poor eyesight, numb feet and hands, insomnia, more dreams, forgetfulness, palpitations and a wandering mind.

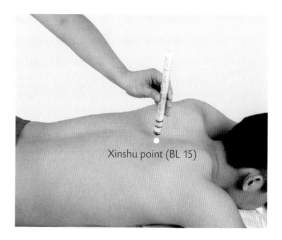

Xinshu point (BL 15)

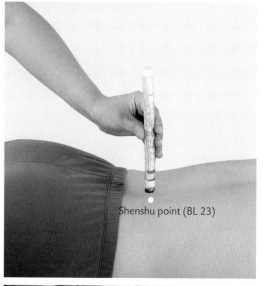

Shenshu point (BL 23)

Sparrow-pecking moxibustion: Apply moxibustion to such points as Pishu, Shenshu, Mingmen, Guanyuan, Neiguan and Zusanli, beginning with those on the back and then the chest and abdomen, first the upper body then the lower body. The practitioner ignites a moxa roll at one side and points it at an acupoint, with the ignited end kept 2 to 3 centimeters from the skin's surface, and moves it up and down, like a sparrow pecking at food. The moxibustion lasts 10 to 15 minutes for each point. Perform the therapy once daily for a 10-day course of treatment with an interval of five days between two courses. This method is suitable for patients suffering from yang deficiency of the spleen and kidneys. Most of these patients suffer from pathogenic cold due to a weak physique, and from continuous diarrhea due to long-term loss of yang qi in the spleen and stomach or weakness of other inner organs impairing the spleen and stomach. The symptoms are characterized either by diarrhea or by constipation.

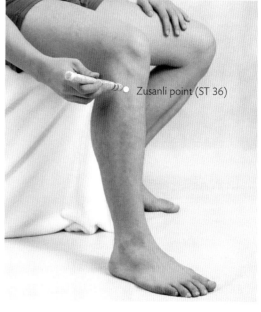

Zusanli point (ST 36)

10. Chronic Hepatitis

Chronic hepatitis is mostly developed from acute viral hepatitis. The body's own immune dysfunction, long-term use of medicine that damages the liver, the body's allergy to medicine, alcohol abuse, lack of a certain enzyme and metabolic disorder can all lead to the occurrence of the disease.

Acupoints of Moxibustion

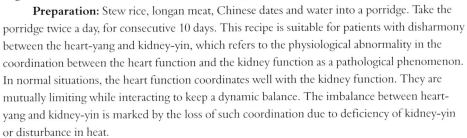

Ganshu point (BL 18)
1.5 cun away from the ninth thoracic spinal process on the inner side of the scapula.

Pishu point (BL 20)
1.5 cun horizontally away from the eleventh thoracic vertebra.

Sanyinjiao point (SP 6)
At the rear edge of the shinbone, 3 cun above the ankle.

Taichong point (LR 3)
On the foot in a notch between the first and second metatarsal bones.

Zusanli point (ST 36)
About 3 cun below the knee on the outer side of the tibia.

Yanglingquan point (GB 34)
On the outer side of the shin in a notch at the front lower part of the fibula.

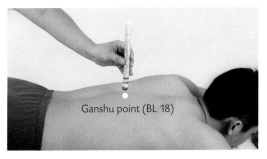

Ganshu point (BL 18)

Moxibustion Method

Mild moxibustion: Moxibustion is applied to such points as Ganshu, Pishu, Yanglingquan, Zusanli, Sanyinjiao, Taichong, beginning with points on the upper body and then moving to those on the lower body. Therapy on points the patient cannot reach can be performed by others. The patient takes a comfortable posture. Ignite one end of a moxa roll and aim it at a point, with the ignited end 3 to 5 centimeters from the skin's surface, until the patient feels warmth but no burning pain. Apply moxibustion to each point for 5 to 7 minutes, until the local skin turns slightly red. Perform the therapy once a day for a 10-day course of treatment with an interval of seven days between two courses.

11. Cholelithiasis

Cholelithiasis is a disease that causes severe abdominal pain, jaundice and fever due to the gallstones produced in the bile duct or gallbladder. The symptoms include varying degrees of pain in the upper abdomen or upper right abdomen, often accompanied by nausea and vomiting in the acute stage.

Cholelithiasis patients should have a light diet, consisting of easily digestible food. Food should be steamed, boiled or stewed. Oil used should be mainly from vegetable sources. Do not eat fried, spicy or irritating food. Eat more vitamin-rich fruits and vegetables. Do appropriate physical exercise to enhance physical fitness and improve the physical ability to resist illness.

Acupoints of Moxibustion

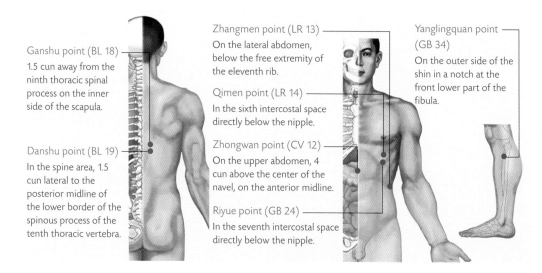

Ganshu point (BL 18)
1.5 cun away from the ninth thoracic spinal process on the inner side of the scapula.

Danshu point (BL 19)
In the spine area, 1.5 cun lateral to the posterior midline of the lower border of the spinous process of the tenth thoracic vertebra.

Zhangmen point (LR 13)
On the lateral abdomen, below the free extremity of the eleventh rib.

Qimen point (LR 14)
In the sixth intercostal space directly below the nipple.

Zhongwan point (CV 12)
On the upper abdomen, 4 cun above the center of the navel, on the anterior midline.

Riyue point (GB 24)
In the seventh intercostal space directly below the nipple.

Yanglingquan point (GB 34)
On the outer side of the shin in a notch at the front lower part of the fibula.

Moxibustion Methods

Mild moxibustion: Moxibustion is applied to such points as Ganshu, Danshu and Yanglingquan, beginning with the points on the upper body and then moving to those on the lower body. The patient should take a comfortable posture. The practitioner ignites one end of a moxa roll and aims it at a point, 3 to 5 centimeters above the skin's surface,

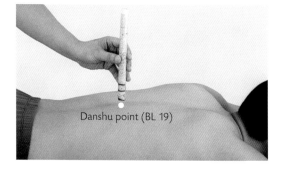

Danshu point (BL 19)

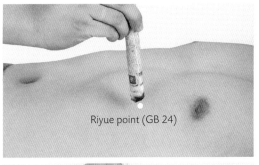
Riyue point (GB 24)

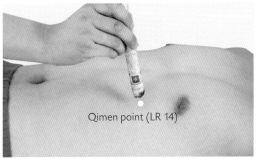
Qimen point (LR 14)

until the patient's local skin feels warm, without the feeling of pain. The patient may try to perform moxibustion of points that she can reach for the best temperature control. Moxibustion lasts 15 to 20 minutes for each point, until the patient feels comfortable and the local skin turns slightly red. Moxibustion is performed once or twice a day for seven times as a course of treatment, with an interval of 3 to 5 days between two courses.

Sparrow-pecking moxibustion: Moxibustion is applied to such points as Riyue, Qimen, Zhangmen and Zhongwan. The patient should take a supine posture. The practitioner ignites a moxa roll at one end and points it at an acupoint, with the ignited end 3 centimeters from the skin, and then holds the stick and moves it up and down, like a sparrow pecking at food, until the patient feels warmth but no pain. Moxibustion lasts five minutes for each point, until the local skin reddens. This is performed once every day, for 10 times as a course of treatment, with an interval of 3 to 5 days between two courses.

12. Peptic Ulcer

Peptic ulcer is a general term for gastric ulcer and duodenal ulcer. Gastric ulcers are mainly found among middle-aged and elderly people, and duodenal ulcers are mainly among young and middle-aged people. The main symptoms are upper abdominal pain, spitting blood and emaciation, which can be accompanied by symptoms such as belching, acid reflux and nausea. Poor diet, environmental factors, psychological factors, diseases, and medications are some causes of peptic ulcers. Moxibustion at related points can improve digestive functions and relieve symptoms.

Patients with peptic ulcers should pay attention to diet regulation, avoid eating coarse grains, crude fibrous vegetables and hard, raw fruits. Do not eat fried food, fatty meat, cream or pungent spices. Choose milk, eggs, lean meat, fish, chicken, tender tofu, noodles, porridge, soft rice and easily digestible vegetables. Have many small meals, chew carefully and swallow slowly. Do not smoke or drink alcohol.

Moxibustion Methods

Swirling moxibustion: Moxibustion is applied to the Danzhong and Zhongwan points. The patient takes a supine posture. The practitioner ignites a moxa roll and points it at an acupoint, about 3 centimeters from the skin, then moves the stick left and right horizontally or circularly above the point, keeping the range of movement just within 3 centimeters, until the local skin feels warm without any pain. Moxibustion lasts 10 to 15 minutes for each point.

This is performed once every day, for 10 times as a course of treatment, with an interval of 3 to 5 days between two courses. When performing moxibustion on a patient with decreased sensitivity, pay attention to skin temperature to avoid burning the skin.

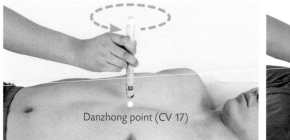
Danzhong point (CV 17)

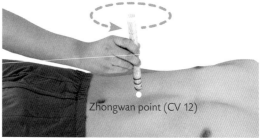
Zhongwan point (CV 12)

Moxibustion with moxa stick roll holder: The patient should take a supine posture. Choose a moxa stick roll holder of the right size and place it on the Guanyuan and Qihai points. Ignite a moxa roll and put it on the mesh, then close the cover to perform moxibustion. The treatment should last 15 to 30 minutes for each point. This is performed once or twice a day, for 10 times as a course of treatment, with an interval of 3 to 5 days between two courses. This therapy is characterized by evenly distributed heat, which makes the patient feel comfortable. During moxibustion, the patient should remain still to avoid bumping the holder and affecting the treatment.

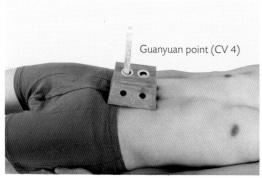
Guanyuan point (CV 4)

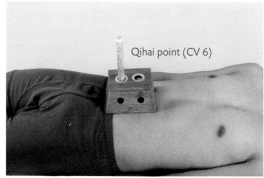
Qihai point (CV 6)

Acupoints of Moxibustion

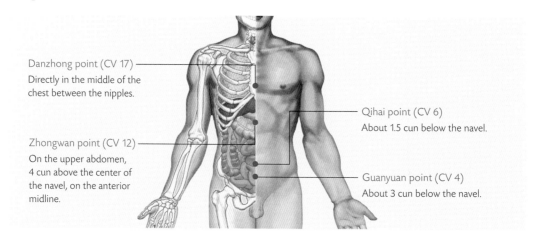

Danzhong point (CV 17)
Directly in the middle of the chest between the nipples.

Zhongwan point (CV 12)
On the upper abdomen, 4 cun above the center of the navel, on the anterior midline.

Qihai point (CV 6)
About 1.5 cun below the navel.

Guanyuan point (CV 4)
About 3 cun below the navel.

13. Chronic Lumbar Muscle Strain

Chronic lumbar muscle strain refers to the chronic injury of lumbosacral muscles, fascia and other soft tissues, which is common among people with chronic lumbago and leg pain. This disease is often related to work environment. It is mainly manifested by recurrent mild to severe waist and back pain, which can be aggravated by fatigue, rainy weather and catching cold. Moxibustion at relevant points can relax muscles, activate meridians, reinforce immunity, and invigorate the liver and kidneys.

    Patients need to correct bad posture and often change their posture during work. Strengthening exercise can help increase the strength of the waist. Prevent sweating when exposed to the wind, so as not to be invaded by pathogenic cold. Overwork can aggravate the condition. Pay attention to local warmth and limit the amount of sexual intercourse. At the same time, traction and other treatments can be used, for example, hot and wet compresses, steaming and washing.

Acupoints of Moxibustion

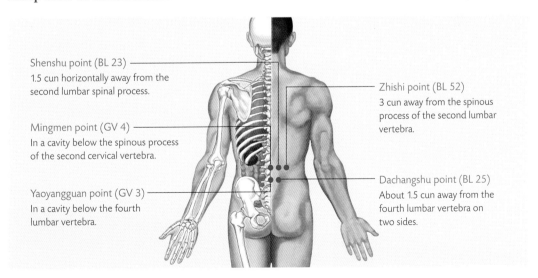

Shenshu point (BL 23)
1.5 cun horizontally away from the second lumbar spinal process.

Mingmen point (GV 4)
In a cavity below the spinous process of the second cervical vertebra.

Yaoyangguan point (GV 3)
In a cavity below the fourth lumbar vertebra.

Zhishi point (BL 52)
3 cun away from the spinous process of the second lumbar vertebra.

Dachangshu point (BL 25)
About 1.5 cun away from the fourth lumbar vertebra on two sides.

Moxibustion Methods

Mild moxibustion: Moxibustion is applied to such points as Ashi, Shenshu, Dachangshu and Yaoyangguan. The patient takes a prone posture. The practitioner, standing one side of the patient, ignites a moxa roll at one end with a match and points it at an acupoint, with the ignited end 3 to 5 centimeters from the skin, until the patient's local skin feels warm without any pain. Moxibustion lasts 15 to 20 minutes for each point, until the patient's local skin turns slightly red in each treatment. Perform once to twice a day for 10 times as a course of treatment, with 3 to 5 days between two courses. The practitioner must be careful to avoid letting the fire contact the skin and to keep falling ashes away from the skin. When applying moxibustion in the winter, be careful to keep the patient warm to avoid catching a cold.

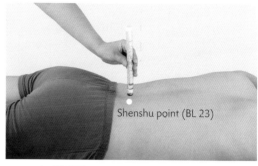

Shenshu point (BL 23)

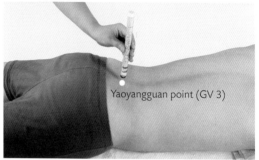

Yaoyangguan point (GV 3)

Moxibustion with moxa box: Moxibustion is applied to Mingmen, Yaoyangguan, Zhishi, Shenshu and other points. Remove the inner box from the moxa box to fill it more than half full with moxa wool. Press the moxa wool surface gently with fingers, as too much compression will affect the moxa burning. Then place the small inner box into the outer tube and ignite moxa wool before closing the top cover.

Cover the targeted skin area with several layers of cloth and place the moxa box on the fabric to start the moxibustion. Perform the therapy for 20 to 30 minutes,

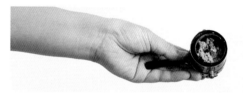

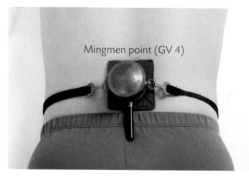

Mingmen point (GV 4)

until local skin turns red and the patient feels comfortable. It is performed once or twice a day, for 10 times as a course of treatment, with an interval of 3 to 5 days between two courses. This technique is simple to implement and produces evenly distributed heat, which is especially suitable for chronic diseases.

14. Periarthritis of the Shoulders

Periarthritis of the shoulders refers to the chronic inflammation of muscles, tendons and other soft tissues in the shoulder area, and the main symptoms are shoulder pain and limited mobility. The disease is most prevalent among people around the age of 50. The incidence is slightly higher in women than men and is more common among manual workers.

According to traditional Chinese medicine, unhealthy muscles and deficiency of qi and blood due to longtime fatigue or catching a cold can lead to periarthritis of the shoulder. Moxibustion at related points can clear meridians, invigorate blood circulation, dispel pathogenic wind and relieve the pain, thus alleviating periarthritis of the shoulder.

Strengthening physical exercise is the most effective way to prevent and treat periarthritis of the shoulder. Persisting in rehabilitation and adherence to exercise can quickly restore shoulder function. In terms of diet, supplement with nutrients to restore physical strength and improve disease resistance. Middle-aged and elderly people should also pay attention to keeping warm and avoid exposing the shoulders to cold. It is necessary to maintain the correct posture and arm-position in daily life and to avoid keeping the same posture for a long time. Constantly change positions to relieve fatigue.

Acupoints of Moxibustion

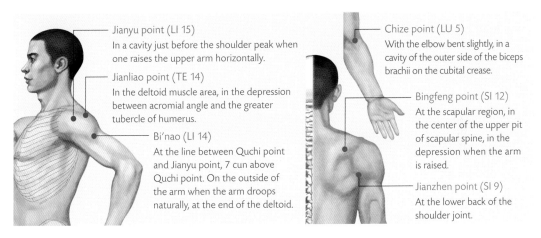

Jianyu point (LI 15)
In a cavity just before the shoulder peak when one raises the upper arm horizontally.

Jianliao point (TE 14)
In the deltoid muscle area, in the depression between acromial angle and the greater tubercle of humerus.

Bi'nao (LI 14)
At the line between Quchi point and Jianyu point, 7 cun above Quchi point. On the outside of the arm when the arm droops naturally, at the end of the deltoid.

Chize point (LU 5)
With the elbow bent slightly, in a cavity of the outer side of the biceps brachii on the cubital crease.

Bingfeng point (SI 12)
At the scapular region, in the center of the upper pit of scapular spine, in the depression when the arm is raised.

Jianzhen point (SI 9)
At the lower back of the shoulder joint.

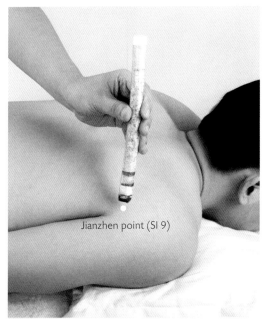

Jianzhen point (SI 9)

Moxibustion Methods

Mild moxibustion: Apply moxibustion to such points as Jianyu, Jianliao, Jianzhen, Bi'nao and Ashi. The patient takes a comfortable posture. Ignite one end of a moxa roll, and hold the ignited head 3 to 5 centimeters from the skin's surface, aiming at an acupoint until the patient's skin around the point feels warmth but no burning pain. Apply moxibustion to each point for 15 to 20 minutes, until the patient's local skin turns slightly red. Perform the therapy once or twice a day for 10 times as a course of treatment, with an interval of three days between two courses. For a patient with decreased sensitivity, the practitioner can place an index finger and a middle finger around the point to feel the temperature, so as not to burn the patient.

Moxibustion with a moxa box:
Moxibustion is applied to the Ashi, Jianyu, Bingfeng and Chize points. The patient takes an appropriate posture. Remove the inner box from the moxa box and place more than half of a box of moxa wool inside. Gently press the moxa wool surface with the fingers, as too much compression will affect the burning of the moxa. Then place the small inner box into the outer box, igniting the moxa wool before closing the top cover. Place several layers of cloth on the related skin area and place the moxa box on top of that to start the moxibustion. Perform the treatment for 10 to 20 minutes, until local skin turns red and the patient feels comfortable. It is performed once or twice a day, for 10 times as a course of treatment,

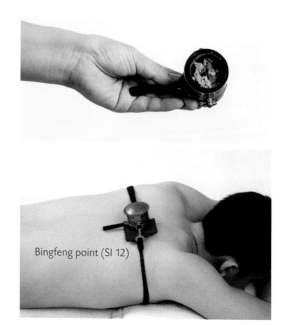

Bingfeng point (SI 12)

with an interval of three days between two courses. This therapy is simple to do and produces balanced distributed heat, with a good therapeutic effect on periarthritis of the shoulder.

15. Cervical Spondylosis

Cervical spondylosis is mainly caused by long-term cervical strain, bone hyperplasia, or cervical intervertebral disc deformation. The main symptoms are neck and shoulder pain, neck stiffness and limited movement. Moxibustion at related points can relax muscles, activate meridians and improve blood circulation, thus treating the pain.

Patients with cervical spondylosis need to correct their bad posture in daily life. While working long hours at a desk, they should periodically get up and move their necks to relieve fatigue. When the weather is cold, pay attention to keeping the neck and waist warm, and avoid negative postures such as shrugging, and bending. In winter, take care to keep the neck and shoulders warm, especially during sleep. Cold irritation can cause a stiff neck, thereby inducing cervical spondylosis and periarthritis of the shoulder. Appropriate exercise helps prevent and treat cervical spondylosis.

Acupoints of Moxibustion

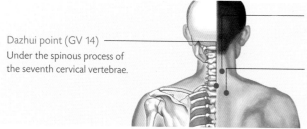

Dazhui point (GV 14)
Under the spinous process of the seventh cervical vertebrae.

Jingbailao point (EX-HN 15)
On the neck, 2 cun above Dazhui point, 1 cun away from the posterior midline.

Dazhu point (BL 11)
In the spine area, 1.5 cun lateral to the posterior midline of the lower border of the spinous process of the first thoracic vertebra.

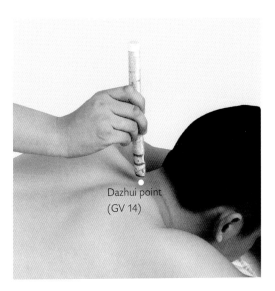

Dazhui point
(GV 14)

Moxibustion Method

Mild moxibustion: Moxibustion is applied to such points as Dazhui, Dazhu, Jingbailao and Ashi. The patient should take a prone posture. The practitioner stands on one side of the patient and ignites a moxa roll at one end, 3 to 5 centimeters from the skin, and points the ignited end at an acupoint to perform moxibustion, until the patient feels warm without the feeling of burning pain. Moxibustion lasts 15 to 20 minutes for each point, until the patient feels comfortable and the local skin turns slightly red. Such moxibustion should be applied once to twice a day for 10 times as a course of treatment, with an interval of 3 to 5 days between two courses.

16. Pain in the Waist and Legs

In mild cases of pain in the waist and legs, discomfort can be relieved after rest but can relapse or worsen with mild trauma or exposure to the cold and dampness. In severe cases, pain will occur in the back of the thighs and the posterior-lateral of the shanks and laterals of the feet, and will be aggravated when turning around, coughing and sneezing, resulting in psoas spasms and scoliosis.

The causes of pain in the waist and legs must be identified; for example, sources include lumbar muscle strain, lumbar disc herniation, visceral disease, inflammation or cancer. Seek treatment of symptoms and do not delay the treatment of this disease.

Acupoints of Moxibustion

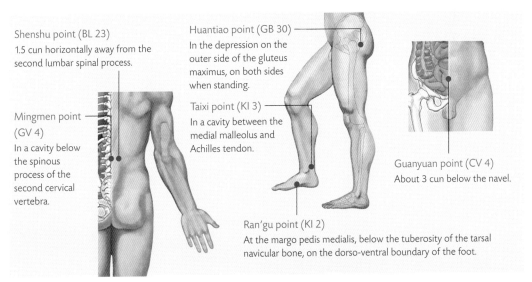

Shenshu point (BL 23)
1.5 cun horizontally away from the second lumbar spinal process.

Mingmen point (GV 4)
In a cavity below the spinous process of the second cervical vertebra.

Huantiao point (GB 30)
In the depression on the outer side of the gluteus maximus, on both sides when standing.

Taixi point (KI 3)
In a cavity between the medial malleolus and Achilles tendon.

Guanyuan point (CV 4)
About 3 cun below the navel.

Ran'gu point (KI 2)
At the margo pedis medialis, below the tuberosity of the tarsal navicular bone, on the dorso-ventral boundary of the foot.

Moxibustion Method

Mild moxibustion: Moxibustion is applied to such points as Shenshu, Mingmen, Huantiao, Guanyuan, Taixi and Ran'gu, beginning with points on the back and then the chest and abdomen, moving from upper to lower body. The patient should take an appropriate position. The practitioner ignites a moxa roll and stands on one side of the patient, pointing the ignited end at an acupoint from 3 to 5 centimeters above the skin's surface, until the patient's skin feels warmth without any pain. Moxibustion lasts 10 to 15 minutes for each point and can be

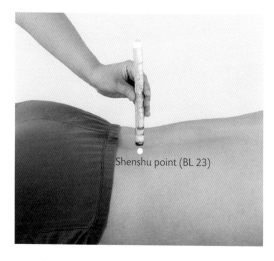

Shenshu point (BL 23)

appropriately extended to 20 to 30 minutes when performing moxibustion to the Shenshu point. This is performed once or twice a day, for 10 times as a course of treatment, with an interval of three days between two courses.

17. Tinnitus

Tinnitus is an abnormal sound sensation produced without any external stimuli and is often a sign of deafness. Tinnitus is a symptom rather than an illness. Patients often feel buzzing or sharp sounds in their ears, making them distracted and restless.

Acupoints of Moxibustion

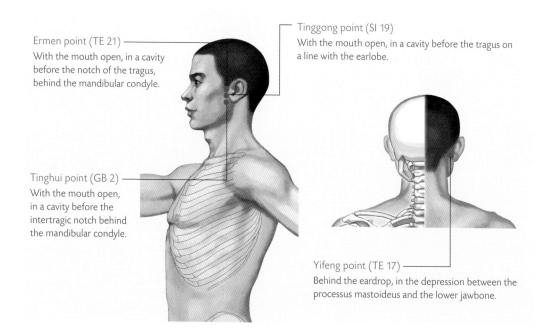

Ermen point (TE 21)
With the mouth open, in a cavity before the notch of the tragus, behind the mandibular condyle.

Tinggong point (SI 19)
With the mouth open, in a cavity before the tragus on a line with the earlobe.

Tinghui point (GB 2)
With the mouth open, in a cavity before the intertragic notch behind the mandibular condyle.

Yifeng point (TE 17)
Behind the eardrop, in the depression between the processus mastoideus and the lower jawbone.

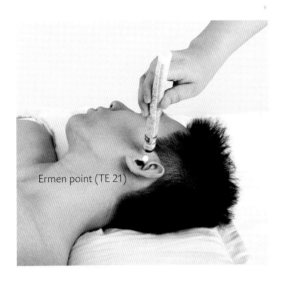

Ermen point (TE 21)

Moxibustion Method

Mild moxibustion: Apply moxibustion to such points as Ermen, Tinggong, Tinghui and Yifeng. The patient should take a comfortable posture. The practitioner, standing on one side of the patient, ignites one end of a moxa roll and points the ignited end at a point, staying 3 to 5 centimeters above the skin's surface, until the patient's local skin feels warm but without pain. Apply moxibustion to each point for 15 to 20 minutes, until the patient feels comfortable and the local skin turns slightly red. Perform once to twice a day for 10 times as a course of treatment, with an interval of 3 to 5 days between two courses.

18. Deafness

Deafness is severe hearing impairment such that the patient can't hear outside sounds. There are many causes of deafness, including heredity, birth trauma, infections, improper use of medicine and poisoning by certain chemicals.

Acupoints of Moxibustion

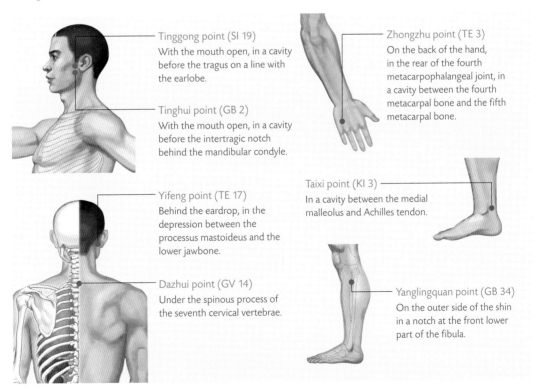

Tinggong point (SI 19)
With the mouth open, in a cavity before the tragus on a line with the earlobe.

Tinghui point (GB 2)
With the mouth open, in a cavity before the intertragic notch behind the mandibular condyle.

Yifeng point (TE 17)
Behind the eardrop, in the depression between the processus mastoideus and the lower jawbone.

Dazhui point (GV 14)
Under the spinous process of the seventh cervical vertebrae.

Zhongzhu point (TE 3)
On the back of the hand, in the rear of the fourth metacarpophalangeal joint, in a cavity between the fourth metacarpal bone and the fifth metacarpal bone.

Taixi point (KI 3)
In a cavity between the medial malleolus and Achilles tendon.

Yanglingquan point (GB 34)
On the outer side of the shin in a notch at the front lower part of the fibula.

Moxibustion Method

Swirling moxibustion: Moxibustion is applied to such points as Tinggong, Tinghui, Yifeng, Dazhui, Zhongzhu, Taixi and Yanglingquan, beginning with points on the head and then the limbs, moving from the upper to lower body. The patient should take an appropriate posture. The practitioner ignites a moxa roll at one end, places it about 3 centimeters above the points, and moves the roll left and right or circularly, within the range of about 3 centimeters, until it brings

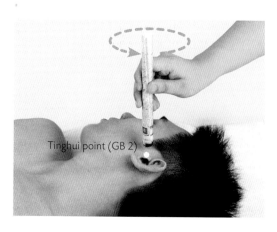

Tinghui point (GB 2)

mild warmth to the skin, without the feeling of burning pain. The moxibustion lasts 10 to 15 minutes for each point. This is performed once every day, for three times as a course of treatment, with an interval of 1 to 2 days between two courses

19. Menopausal Syndrome

Menopausal syndrome is a series of symptoms caused by decreased levels of estrogen, such as menstrual changes, facial flushing, palpitations, insomnia, fatigue, depression, emotional instability, irritability and difficulty concentrating.

It is necessary to correctly understand the arrival of menopause and make full preparations mentally. Have peaceful emotions, be positive and optimistic about life, avoid vexation and complaints and make a good psychological adjustment. Pay attention to reasonable diet and nourishment; eat low-calorie, low-fat, low-sugar, high-protein and high-vitamin food, ensuring intake of appropriate inorganic salts. Adhering to a proper physical exercise routine can not only enhance physical fitness, but also make people feel comfortable. Maintain a proper balance between work and rest to ensure adequate sleep. If the condition is severe, appropriate medical treatment can be used.

Moxibustion Method

Mild moxibustion: Moxibustion is applied to such points as Shenshu, Sanyinjiao, Zusanli, Zhongji, Zigong, Taixi, Zhishi, Taichong and Ganshu, beginning with the points on the waist and back and then those on the chest and abdomen, moving from the upper to lower body. The patient may have others perform moxibustion of points that are inaccessible to her, and perform moxibustion herself on the ones she can reach, allowing better control of temperature and location. Ignite one end of a moxa roll and point the ignited end at a point, staying

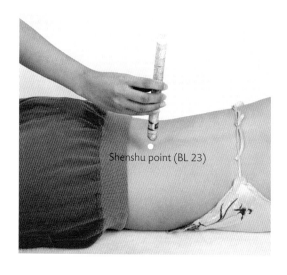

Shenshu point (BL 23)

3 to 5 centimeters above the skin. Moxibustion lasts 10 to 20 minutes for each point, until the patient feels comfortable and the local skin turns slightly red. Such treatment should be given daily for a 10-day course of treatment with an interval of 3 to 5 days between two courses.

1. Lotus Seed Porridge with Lilies

Ingredients: 1.1 ounces each of lotus seeds, lilies and rice.

      Preparation: Stew porridge with lotus seeds, lilies and rice. Eat this porridge every morning and evening. It is indicated for palpitations, sleeplessness, delirium, forgetfulness, limb weakness and rough skin before and after menopause.

2. Date Porridge

Ingredients: 1.1 ounces of spina date seeds, 2.1 ounces of rice.

      Preparation: Wash spina date seeds, decoct them with water. Take the juice and cook it with rice into porridge. Eat it once a day for a 10-day course of treatment. This recipe is indicated for mental disorders, unpredictable temper, lusterless complexion and poor appetite in menopause.

Acupoints of Moxibustion

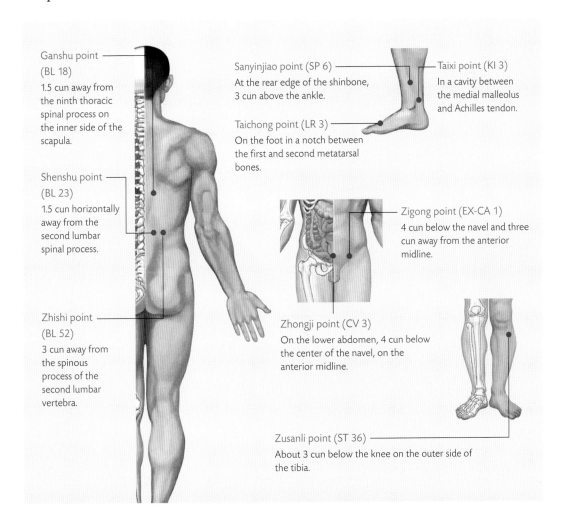

Ganshu point (BL 18)
1.5 cun away from the ninth thoracic spinal process on the inner side of the scapula.

Shenshu point (BL 23)
1.5 cun horizontally away from the second lumbar spinal process.

Zhishi point (BL 52)
3 cun away from the spinous process of the second lumbar vertebra.

Sanyinjiao point (SP 6)
At the rear edge of the shinbone, 3 cun above the ankle.

Taichong point (LR 3)
On the foot in a notch between the first and second metatarsal bones.

Taixi point (KI 3)
In a cavity between the medial malleolus and Achilles tendon.

Zigong point (EX-CA 1)
4 cun below the navel and three cun away from the anterior midline.

Zhongji point (CV 3)
On the lower abdomen, 4 cun below the center of the navel, on the anterior midline.

Zusanli point (ST 36)
About 3 cun below the knee on the outer side of the tibia.

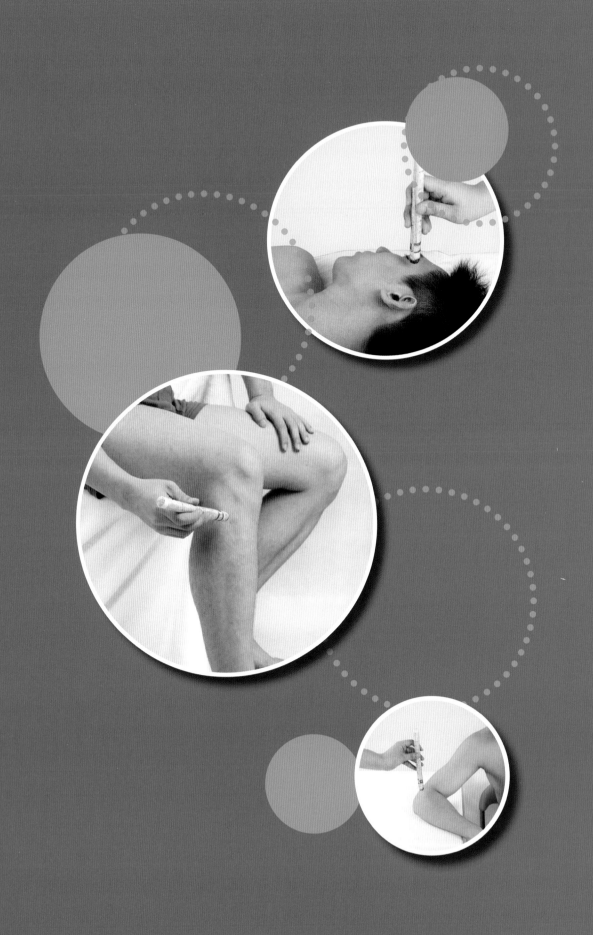

CHAPTER FIVE
Moxibustion Therapy for Health Care

Moxibustion can not only cure diseases, but also provide health care. When one is in poor health and experiencing fatigue, restlessness, uncomfortable emotions and other painful conditions, one can use moxibustion to relieve symptoms, regulate emotions and avoid illness.

1. Preventing against Colds

The cold is a common illness, but not unpreventable. Regular precautions to improve the immune system, enhance lung functions and drive exogenous pathogenic factors out can help one avoid catching cold. In the seasons when one can easily catch a cold, moxibustion at relevant points once a day or every other day can also help prevent colds.

Enhancing immunity is the key to cold prevention. In terms of diet, eat less spicy and irritating food, and eat more fresh fruits and vegetables to increase vitamins E and C, which can effectively improve immunity. Drinking a large amount of water every day can remove viruses from the body through the circulation of body fluids. Soak the feet in warm water for at least 15 minutes before going to sleep every night. Ensure adequate sleep. Thirty to forty minutes of daily aerobic exercise can enhance the body's ability to resist colds.

Acupoints of Moxibustion

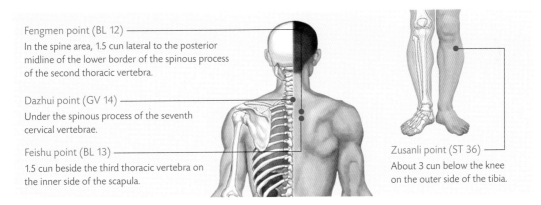

Fengmen point (BL 12)
In the spine area, 1.5 cun lateral to the posterior midline of the lower border of the spinous process of the second thoracic vertebra.

Dazhui point (GV 14)
Under the spinous process of the seventh cervical vertebrae.

Feishu point (BL 13)
1.5 cun beside the third thoracic vertebra on the inner side of the scapula.

Zusanli point (ST 36)
About 3 cun below the knee on the outer side of the tibia.

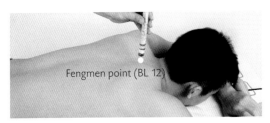

Fengmen point (BL 12)

Moxibustion Methods

Mild moxibustion: Moxibustion is applied first to the Fengmen point and then Zusanli. The patient takes an appropriate position. The practitioner ignites one end of a moxa roll and points the ignited end at a point,

3 to 5 centimeters above the skin's surface, until the person receiving moxibustion feels warmth without pain. Moxibustion lasts 20 to 30 minutes for each point, until the skin turns slightly red. Perform once every day or every other day for five times as a course of treatment, with an interval of three days between two courses. The patient is suggested to perform moxibustion of Zusanli point by himself to better control the temperature. This therapy can eliminate or reduce cold symptoms.

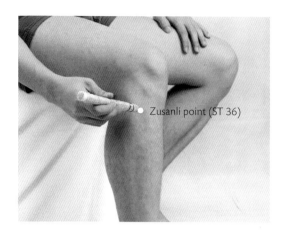

Zusanli point (ST 36)

Moxibustion with moxa stick roll holder: Apply moxibustion to the Dazhui, Fengmen and Feishu points. After the patient takes an appropriate posture, choose a large-sized moxa box, and place it on the points for moxibustion. Ignite the moxa roll and put it on the mesh, and then close the cover to perform moxibustion. Moxibustion lasts 20 to 30 minutes for each point. Perform once every two or three days for five times as a course of treatment, with an interval of three days between two courses. This method is characterized by balanced distributed heat, which makes the person receiving moxibustion feel comfortable. It can prevent one from catching a cold.

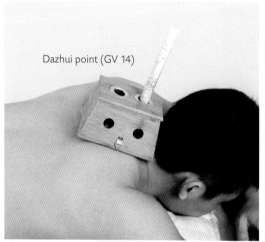

Dazhui point (GV 14)

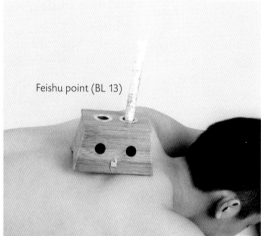

Feishu point (BL 13)

When one feels that she is about to catch a cold, some helper methods can be used to prevent the cold.

1. Nasal irrigation: Every morning and evening, washing the nasal cavity with saline water can excrete contaminants from the nasal cavity, preventing the virus from multiplying in the nasal cavity and inducing a cold.

2. Ginger tea: Take an appropriate amount of brown sugar, ginger and black tea, and boil them before drinking. Drink once or twice a day to help prevent a cold.

3. Honey water: Drinking honey water once every morning and evening can effectively enhance the body's immunity and prevent disease.

2. Strengthening the Spleen and Stomach

The spleen and stomach are the main organs of the digestive system and have the function of digesting food and absorbing nutrients. If the functions of the spleen and stomach are normal, then qi and blood are sufficient, and the body is healthy; otherwise, if qi and blood are deficient, the body will be weak. Moxibustion at relevant points can increase the temperature of the spleen and stomach meridians, expel the cold, enhance the spleen and stomach functions, and promote food digestion and absorption, as well as the gastrointestinal tract's metabolizing function to achieve optimal health.

People with spleen and stomach disorders must pay attention to diet regulation: They should eat less fried food, pickled food, and raw, cold and irritating food. They should mainly eat low-fat and light food, eat a fixed amount regularly and not eat or drink too much. The temperature of meals should not be too hot or too cold to avoid irritating the intestines and stomach. Patients should chew carefully and swallow slowly when eating, and avoid smoking or drinking liquor. They should maintain a proper balance between work and rest, and exercise regularly to increase the functions of inner organs and enhance immunity.

Acupoints of Moxibustion

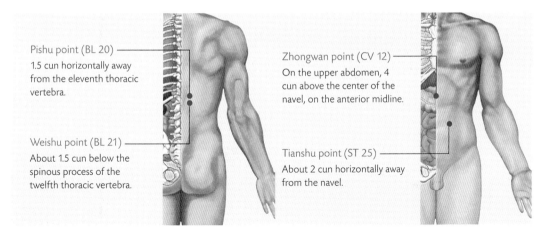

Pishu point (BL 20)
1.5 cun horizontally away from the eleventh thoracic vertebra.

Weishu point (BL 21)
About 1.5 cun below the spinous process of the twelfth thoracic vertebra.

Zhongwan point (CV 12)
On the upper abdomen, 4 cun above the center of the navel, on the anterior midline.

Tianshu point (ST 25)
About 2 cun horizontally away from the navel.

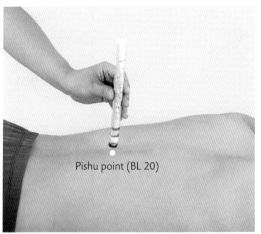

Pishu point (BL 20)

Moxibustion Method

Mild moxibustion: Moxibustion is applied to the Pishu, Weishu, Zhongwan, Tianshu and other points, beginning with points on the waist and back and then moving on to those on the chest and abdomen. The patient should take an appropriate posture, with the skin above the acupoints exposed. The practitioner ignites a moxa roll and points the ignited end at a point, 3 to 5 centimeters from the skin's surface, until the person receiving moxibustion feels warmth without pain. Apply moxibustion to each point for 10 to 20 minutes, until the skin turns slightly red. Perform the therapy once a day or once every other day for 10 times as a course of treatment, with an interval of 3 to 5 days between two courses. If the patient has reduced sensation, the practitioner can place an index and a middle finger around the point to feel the temperature, so as not to burn the patient's skin.

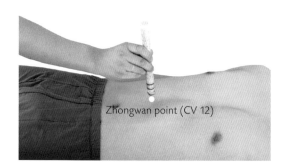
Zhongwan point (CV 12)

Mung Bean Porridge

Ingredients: 3.5 ounces of green beans, 5.3 ounces of rice, 0.5 ounce of sugar.

Preparation: Wash the green beans and rice, put them into a pot and add an appropriate amount of water. Boil slowly into a porridge over low heat. Add sugar when the porridge is cooked. Eat as a main course in the morning and evening every day. This recipe is indicated for the disorder of the spleen and stomach, loss of appetite and weak digestion.

3. Enhancing Immunity

Immunity is the human body's defense mechanism, and drives the body's physiological response to identify and eliminate unwanted biological invasions. If immunity is strong, the body will be healthy and less susceptible to disease; weak immunity increases the probability of illness, as the body is more vulnerable to viruses and bacteria. Many factors can decrease immunity, malnutrition, prolonged illness, over-fatigue and bad mood. Applying moxibustion at related points can improve the functions of inner organs and improve immunity.

To improve immunity, diet and exercise are key. Eat more food rich in protein, vitamins and minerals, such as cucumbers, tomatoes, kelp, mushrooms, yogurt and radishes. Eat less food high in fat and sugar, do not smoke, and drink less liquor. Aim for 30 to 40 minutes of daily exercise like running, swimming or *taijiquan*, which can effectively enhance the physical resistance. Cultivate a variety of interests, stay energetic, and learn to reduce pressure and keep a positive mood.

Acupoints of Moxibustion

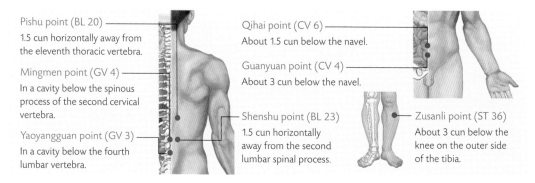

Pishu point (BL 20)
1.5 cun horizontally away from the eleventh thoracic vertebra.

Mingmen point (GV 4)
In a cavity below the spinous process of the second cervical vertebra.

Yaoyangguan point (GV 3)
In a cavity below the fourth lumbar vertebra.

Qihai point (CV 6)
About 1.5 cun below the navel.

Guanyuan point (CV 4)
About 3 cun below the navel.

Shenshu point (BL 23)
1.5 cun horizontally away from the second lumbar spinal process.

Zusanli point (ST 36)
About 3 cun below the knee on the outer side of the tibia.

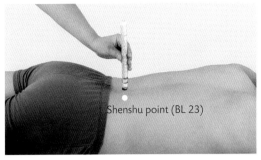

Shenshu point (BL 23)

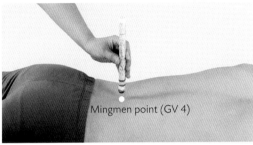

Mingmen point (GV 4)

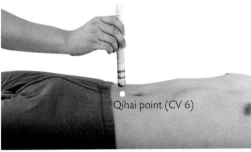

Qihai point (CV 6)

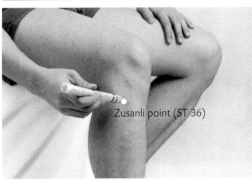

Zusanli point (ST 36)

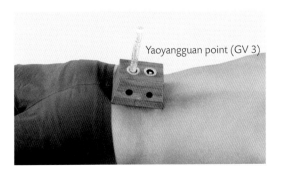

Yaoyangguan point (GV 3)

Moxibustion Methods

Mild moxibustion: Moxibustion is applied to the Feishu, Shenshu, Mingmen and Zusanli points, moving from points on the upper to lower body. The patient takes an appropriate posture, and the practitioner ignites a moxa roll at one end and points the ignited end at a point, 3 to 5 centimeters above the skin's surface, until the skin of the person receiving moxibustion feels warmth but no pain. The patient can perform moxibustion of the Zusanli point herself for better temperature control. Apply moxibustion to each point for 15 to 20 minutes, until the patient's local skin turns slightly red. Perform the therapy once or twice a day for 10 times as a course of treatment, with an interval of 3 to 5 days between two courses. During moxibustion, the practitioner should be careful to avoid burning the skin with falling ash.

Swirling moxibustion: Moxibustion is applied to the Qihai, Guanyuan, Zusanli and Shenshu points, beginning with points on the waist and back and then those on the chest and abdomen, moving from points on the upper to lower body. The person receiving moxibustion should take an appropriate posture. The practitioner stands on one side of the patient, ignites a moxa roll at one end and points the ignited end at an acupoint, 3 to 5 centimeters above the skin. The practitioner holds the roll and moves it left and right or circularly, within the range of about 3 centimeters, until the person receiving moxibustion feels warmth but no pain. Moxibustion lasts 10 to 15 minutes for each point, until the skin turns slightly red. Perform the therapy once or twice a day, for 10 times as a course of treatment, with an interval of 3 to 5 days between two courses.

Moxibustion with moxa stick roll holder: Moxibustion is applied to the Shenshu, Mingmen, Yaoyangguan, Qihai and Guanyuan points. The person receiving moxibustion should take an appropriate posture. Choose a large-sized holder and place it on the point for moxibustion. Ignite a moxa roll and put it on the mesh, then close the cover to perform moxibustion. Moxibustion lasts 15 to 30 minutes for each point. Perform the therapy once or twice a day, for 10 times as a course of treatment, with an interval of 3 to 5 days between two

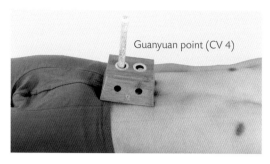

Guanyuan point (CV 4)

courses. This method is characterized by balanced distributed heat, which will make the person receiving moxibustion feel comfortable.

4. Reinforcing Kidney Function

By filtering the blood and producing urine, kidneys maintain the human body's internal environmental stability and enable normal metabolism, and their proper functioning is closely related to overall health. If kidney essence is sufficient, then one will be full of energy and enjoy quick thinking, a strong memory, strong bones and muscles and physical agility. Otherwise, symptoms such as dizziness, palpitations, shortness of breath, fatigue, and soreness and weakness of waist and knees may occur. Applying moxibustion at relevant points can reinforce the kidney function and build up health.

In terms of diet, eggs, oysters, shrimp and quail are the top choices for the care of kidneys. Keep warm in the winter and do not expose the body to cold. Drink plenty of water and do not hold back urine, as this can cause bacteria to infect the kidneys. Increase exercise to help remove toxins from the body and improve kidney function.

Acupoints of Moxibustion

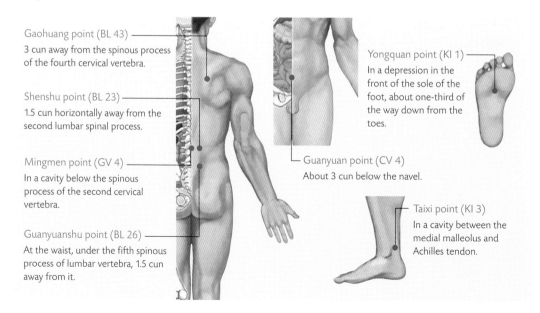

Gaohuang point (BL 43)
3 cun away from the spinous process of the fourth cervical vertebra.

Shenshu point (BL 23)
1.5 cun horizontally away from the second lumbar spinal process.

Mingmen point (GV 4)
In a cavity below the spinous process of the second cervical vertebra.

Guanyuanshu point (BL 26)
At the waist, under the fifth spinous process of lumbar vertebra, 1.5 cun away from it.

Yongquan point (KI 1)
In a depression in the front of the sole of the foot, about one-third of the way down from the toes.

Guanyuan point (CV 4)
About 3 cun below the navel.

Taixi point (KI 3)
In a cavity between the medial malleolus and Achilles tendon.

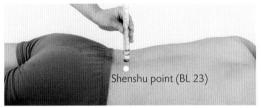
Shenshu point (BL 23)

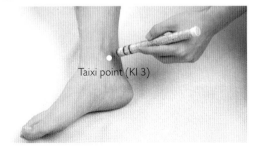
Taixi point (KI 3)

Moxibustion Method

Mild moxibustion: Moxibustion is applied to the Shenshu, Taixi, Mingmen, Guanyuan, Yongquan, Gaohuang and Guanyuanshu points, beginning with points on the waist and back and then moving to those on the chest and abdomen, working the points from the upper to lower body. The person receiving moxibustion should take an appropriate posture. The practitioner ignites a moxa roll at one end and points the ignited end at a point, 3 to 5 centimeters above the skin's surface, until the person receiving moxibustion feels warm, without the feeling of pain. Moxibustion lasts 10 to 20 minutes for each point, until the skin turns slightly red. Perform moxibustion once every two or three days for 10 times as a course of treatment, with an interval of 3 to 5 days between two courses.

5. Nourishing the Heart and Calming the Nerves

If people are disconcerted, there will be symptoms such as palpitations, forgetfulness, insomnia, absent-mindedness, dreaminess, nocturnal emissions, aphtha of the mouth and tongue, and dry stools. These symptoms are mostly caused by deficiency of blood in the heart. Applying moxibustion at related points can activate blood circulation, nourish myocardium, improve heart function, tranquilize and allay excitement, and make people energetic, calm and quick-thinking. Regular moxibustion can maintain good health and increase longevity.

Regularly eat food that helps to calm the mind, such as lotus seeds, longan, Chinese dates, lily, milk and millet. Eat more fresh fruits and vegetables to supplement the body's nutrients. Eat fewer spicy and irritating foods, including pepper, coffee, strong tea. Avoid alcohol and tobacco. Avoid staying up late to ensure adequate sleep and improve sleep quality. Regularly exercise to promote blood circulation, discharge toxins from the body and improve nerve functions. Stay happy and avoid stress and emotional instability.

Acupoints of Moxibustion

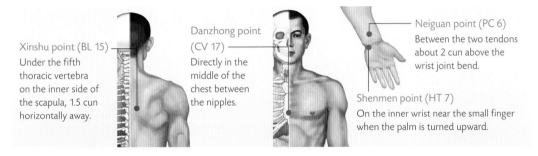

Xinshu point (BL 15)
Under the fifth thoracic vertebra on the inner side of the scapula, 1.5 cun horizontally away.

Danzhong point (CV 17)
Directly in the middle of the chest between the nipples.

Neiguan point (PC 6)
Between the two tendons about 2 cun above the wrist joint bend.

Shenmen point (HT 7)
On the inner wrist near the small finger when the palm is turned upward.

Moxibustion Method

Mild moxibustion: Moxibustion is applied to such points as Neiguan, Xinshu, Shenmen and Danzhong, beginning with points on the waist and back and then moving on to those on the chest and abdomen. The person receiving moxibustion should take an appropriate posture, with the skin above the points exposed. The practitioner, standing on one side of the patient, ignites a moxa roll at one end and points the ignited end at a point, 3 to 5 centimeters above the skin's surface, until the treated area feels warm, without the feeling of pain. Moxibustion lasts 5 to 10 minutes for each point, until the skin turns slightly red. The moxibustion is given once a day and repeated for 20 to 30 days for a course of treatment with a 7- to 10-day interval between two courses.

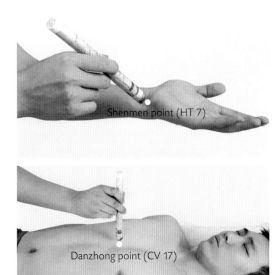

Shenmen point (HT 7)

Danzhong point (CV 17)

1. Lily Honey Porridge

Ingredients: 3.5 ounces of lilies, 3.5 ounces of rice, appropriate amount of honey.

Preparation: After lilies and rice are cooked into porridge, add honey. Drink before going to bed at night, to nourish the mind; or soak roses with water and add honey for a recipe that can soothe the liver and ease the mind.

2. Lotus Seed Porridge

Ingredients: 1.1 ounces of lotus seeds, 3.5 ounces of rice.

Preparation: First grind lotus seeds into a powder, and add this to the rice after boiling it into porridge. Mix before eating. This dish serves to reinforce spleen functions, replenish the kidneys, nourish the heart and calm the mind.

6. Nourishing the Brain and Benefiting Intelligence

The brain is the most precise organ in the human body, and nourishing it is the first defense against decline in brain functions. If the brain functions decline, there will be memory loss, slowed reaction time, lack of concentration, loss of appetite, dizziness, and other symptoms. Moxibustion at related points can dredge meridians and invigorate qi and blood, increase blood flow to the brain, and regulate cranial nerves, thereby stimulating the spirit, eliminating fatigue, improving memory and helping to maintain a clear head.

Frequent intake of food beneficial to intelligence and the brain, such as walnuts, soybeans, longan, black sesame seeds, wolfberry fruit and fish, can promote brain development and enhance memory. Adhering to physical exercise, like running, playing ball games, swimming, or *taijiquan*, can promote blood circulation and keep people active. Stay happy, learn to ease stress, maintain an optimistic attitude toward life, and use the brain more frequently to keep your brain active.

Acupoints of Moxibustion

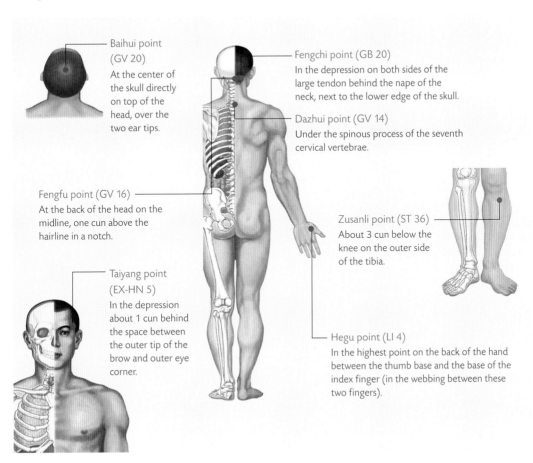

Baihui point (GV 20)
At the center of the skull directly on top of the head, over the two ear tips.

Fengchi point (GB 20)
In the depression on both sides of the large tendon behind the nape of the neck, next to the lower edge of the skull.

Dazhui point (GV 14)
Under the spinous process of the seventh cervical vertebrae.

Fengfu point (GV 16)
At the back of the head on the midline, one cun above the hairline in a notch.

Zusanli point (ST 36)
About 3 cun below the knee on the outer side of the tibia.

Taiyang point (EX-HN 5)
In the depression about 1 cun behind the space between the outer tip of the brow and outer eye corner.

Hegu point (LI 4)
In the highest point on the back of the hand between the thumb base and the base of the index finger (in the webbing between these two fingers).

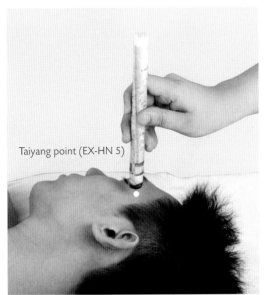

Taiyang point (EX-HN 5)

Moxibustion Method

Mild moxibustion: Moxibustion is applied to the Baihui, Taiyang, Fengchi, Fengfu, Dazhui, Hegu and Zusanli points, beginning with points on the head and face and then those on the limbs, moving from the upper to lower body. The person receiving moxibustion should take an appropriate posture. The practitioner ignites a moxa roll at one end and points the ignited end at an acupoint, 3 to 5 centimeters above the skin's surface, until the person receiving moxibustion feels warmth but no pain. Moxibustion lasts 10 to 15 minutes for each point, once every two or three days, and 1 to 3 months for a course of treatment with an interval of 3 to 5 days between two courses. The hair should be parted to both sides before performing moxibustion to points covered by the hair.

1. Fungus Scrambled Eggs

Ingredients: 7.1 ounces of eggs, 8.8 ounces of fungus (soaked in water), appropriate amount of salt.

Preparation: Wash the soaked and swollen fungus and drain for future use. Beat the eggs into a bowl and stir well. Heat the pan. Add an appropriate amount of cooking oil. After the pan is slightly heated, add eggs to the pan and remove them when they are cooked. Add enough cooking oil to the pan and add the fungus, fry for a few minutes, then add eggs, salt and other seasonings before eating. Lecithin and vitamin B2 in eggs play a significant role in the nerve system and human growth. After being digested, lecithin will release choline to promote the cerebral growth and improve memory.

2. Fried Golden Needle Mushrooms

Ingredients: 7.1 ounces of golden needle mushrooms, 7.1 ounces of cucumbers, 5.3 ounces of bamboo shoots, appropriate amount of ginger, cooking wine, salt and monosodium glutamate.

Preparation: Wash the golden needle mushrooms, cut off the stalks, wash and slice cucumbers and bamboo shoots; put golden needle mushrooms and bamboo shoots into boiled water for a while and then drain them. Pour cooking oil into the pot. After it is heated, stir-fry the ginger, add cooking wine, monosodium glutamate and salt. Pick out the ginger, add the mushrooms, cucumber slices and bamboo shoot slices and fry them well, then top with sesame oil. Golden needle mushrooms have quite comprehensive elements of amino acid necessary for the human body, particularly rich in lysine and arginine, with a fairly high content of zinc, producing the desirable effect of reinforcing intelligence; these especially important for children's height and intelligence development.

7. Nourishing the Liver to Improve Eyesight

Eyes are the foremost of the five sensory organs. They play such a vital role that they're often referred to as "the windows of the soul." Eyes have a close relationship with the liver, and normal vision can be maintained only when eyes are nourished by liver blood. Moxibustion at related points can enhance liver functions and dredge meridians, thus protecting eyes and restoring eyesight. Moxibustion can also prevent and cure various eye diseases, as well as protect the eyes at any age.

Scientifically planning the diet and eating more fish roe, fish liver, fish meat and so on can help keep the eyes healthy. Eat liver-nourishing foods regularly, including melon seeds, sweet potatoes, soybeans and Chinese dates. Avoid overuse of the eyes, and do eye exercises regularly. Maintain a good work-life balance, and avoid staying up late. Drinking less alcohol, as heavy drinking causes the greatest damage to the liver. Moderate exercise promotes blood circulation and removes toxins from the body. Pay attention to regulating the emotions and keeping calm to reduce liver damage as much as possible.

Moxibustion Method

Mild moxibustion: Moxibustion is applied to such points as Quchi, Ganshu, Hegu, Taiyang, Yangbai and Sibai, starting with the points on the head and face and then those on the limbs, moving from points on the upper body to those on the lower body. The person receiving moxibustion should take an appropriate posture. The practitioner, standing on one side of the patient, ignites a moxa roll at one end and points the ignited end at a point, 3 to 5 centimeters above the skin's surface, until the skin feels warm, without the feeling of pain. Moxibustion lasts 10 minutes for each point, until the skin turns slightly red. Moxibustion is performed once or twice each week for four times as a course of treatment, with an interval of one week between two courses. When applying moxibustion to facial points, be careful not to let falling ash burn the skin.

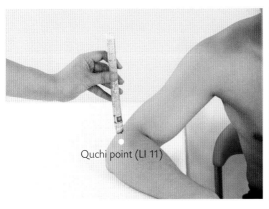

Quchi point (LI 11)

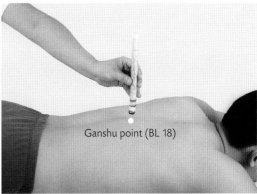

Ganshu point (BL 18)

Acupoints of Moxibustion

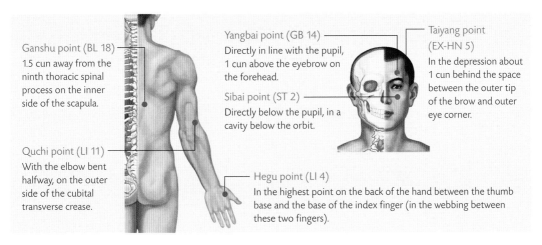

Ganshu point (BL 18)
1.5 cun away from the ninth thoracic spinal process on the inner side of the scapula.

Quchi point (LI 11)
With the elbow bent halfway, on the outer side of the cubital transverse crease.

Yangbai point (GB 14)
Directly in line with the pupil, 1 cun above the eyebrow on the forehead.

Sibai point (ST 2)
Directly below the pupil, in a cavity below the orbit.

Hegu point (LI 4)
In the highest point on the back of the hand between the thumb base and the base of the index finger (in the webbing between these two fingers).

Taiyang point (EX-HN 5)
In the depression about 1 cun behind the space between the outer tip of the brow and outer eye corner.

Chrysanthemum Porridge
Ingredients: 1.8 ounces of rice, 0.4 ounce of chrysanthemum, 1.1 ounces of rock candy.
Preparation: First cook rice and rock candy in 17.1 ounces of water until the rice is ready and the soup becomes thick. Add chrysanthemum powder (chrysanthemums dried in sunlight and ground). Cook for a few minutes on low heat. Turn off the heat after the porridge is thick and let the mixture rest covered in the pot for five minutes before eating. Eat twice a day, warming the porridge slightly before serving. This porridge helps clear heat, clear the liver and brighten the eyes, and is suitable for dealing with headache, hot eyes, dizziness caused by high blood pressure and cold due to wind-heat, as well as swelling and eye pain caused by wind-heat in liver meridians. People with deficiency of qi and stomach cold or reduced appetite with diarrhea should eat less of this porridge.

8. Health Care for Middle-Aged and Elderly People

As people move through mid-life and then old age, their body functions gradually decline, and various diseases can follow. Therefore, it is very important to strengthen health care. Moxibustion at relevant points can dredge and activate the meridians, invigorate the circulation of qi and blood, and nourish the liver and kidneys, thus helping to regulate blood pressure, reduce blood fat, prevent and cure diseases and delay aging.

Middle-aged and elderly people should have a reasonable diet, consume appropriate calories and maintain a normal weight. They should be sure to get enough high-quality protein, and often eat eggs, milk and bean products. It's important to control the consumption of animal fat, keep the diet light and ensure the intake of various minerals and trace elements. Eat plenty of fruits and vegetables to ensure adequate vitamin intake, and take an appropriate calcium supplement. Do not smoke or drink liquor. Maintain a proper balance between work and rest, do not overwork and ensure adequate sleep. Do more aerobic exercise, such as walking, *taijiquan* and dancing. Develop interests and hobbies, for example calligraphy and painting, to calm the mind and prolong life.

Acupoints of Moxibustion

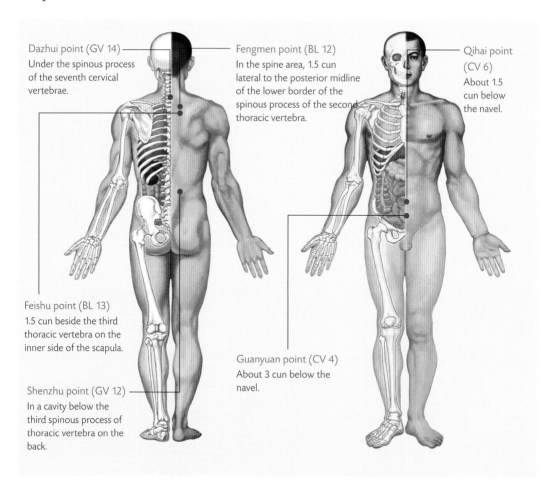

Dazhui point (GV 14)
Under the spinous process of the seventh cervical vertebrae.

Fengmen point (BL 12)
In the spine area, 1.5 cun lateral to the posterior midline of the lower border of the spinous process of the second thoracic vertebra.

Qihai point (CV 6)
About 1.5 cun below the navel.

Feishu point (BL 13)
1.5 cun beside the third thoracic vertebra on the inner side of the scapula.

Guanyuan point (CV 4)
About 3 cun below the navel.

Shenzhu point (GV 12)
In a cavity below the third spinous process of thoracic vertebra on the back.

Moxibustion Method

Mild moxibustion: Moxibustion is applied to such points as Qihai, Feishu, Fengmen, Dazhui, Shenshu and Guanyuan, beginning with points on the waist and back and then moving to those on the chest and abdomen. The person receiving moxibustion should take an appropriate posture, with points for moxibustion exposed. The practitioner ignites one end of a moxa roll and points the ignited end at an acupoint, 3 to 5 centimeters above the skin's surface, until the person receiving moxibustion feels warmth but no pain. Apply moxibustion to each point for 10 to 20 minutes, until the skin turns red. Perform it once daily or once every other day, and the course of treatment is not limited.

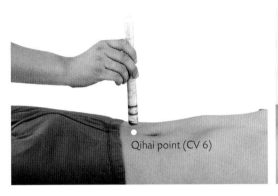

Qihai point (CV 6)

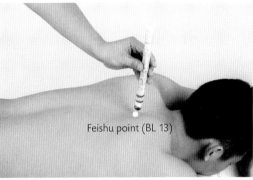

Feishu point (BL 13)

Middle-aged and elderly people can often massage the Hegu, Neiguan and Zusanli points. These three points are health-care points that can regulate qi and blood and prevent and cure diseases. However, in the process of massage, proper force and methods should be used. The force applied should be moderate; too much pressure can be uncomfortable, but too little will fail to produce any stimulating effect.

9. Health Care for Young Adults

Young adult generally refers to people between the ages of 18 and 39. People this age are under heavy pressure in terms of study, daily life and work. Many people are in a sub-health state and need health care. Moxibustion at relevant points can adjust qi and blood, enhance the functions of inner organs, nourish yin essence and improve the body's immunity, thus improving energy, strengthening qi, blood, muscles and bones, and also relieving work pressure.

Though having the best physical condition at this stage, young adults should not over-consume their energy, exhausting the body and spirit. They should pay attention to a proper balance of work and rest, and avoid overwork or staying up late. They should maintain a normal daily life schedule and a healthful diet, avoiding overly fatty, sweet or spicy food. It is also important to eat more fruits and vegetables, smoke less and drink less alcohol. They should also exercise regularly to remove toxins from the body, promote blood circulation and enhance body resistance. Striving to stay happy and learning to relieve stress are also crucial to health.

Acupoints of Moxibustion

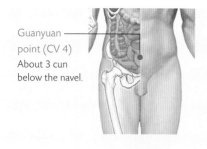

Guanyuan point (CV 4)
About 3 cun below the navel.

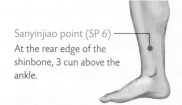

Sanyinjiao point (SP 6)
At the rear edge of the shinbone, 3 cun above the ankle.

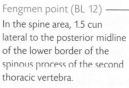

Fengmen point (BL 12)
In the spine area, 1.5 cun lateral to the posterior midline of the lower border of the spinous process of the second thoracic vertebra.

Feishu point (BL 13)
1.5 cun beside the third thoracic vertebra on the inner side of the scapula.

Shenshu point (BL 23)
1.5 cun horizontally away from the second lumbar spinal process.

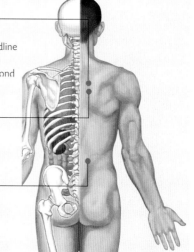

Moxibustion Methods

Mild moxibustion: Moxibustion is applied to such points as Guanyuan, Shenshu, Sanyinjiao, Fengmen and Feishu, beginning with points on the waist and back and then moving to those on the chest and abdomen, working from the upper to lower body. The person receiving moxibustion should take an appropriate posture. The practitioner ignites one end of a moxa roll and aims the ignited end at a point, 3 to 5 centimeters above the skin's surface, until the person receiving moxibustion feels warmth without pain. Apply moxibustion to each point for 10 to 20 minutes, until the skin turns red. Perform it once every 2 to 3 days for a one-month course of treatment with an interval of 3 to 5 days between two courses.

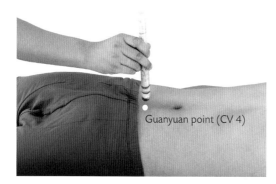

Guanyuan point (CV 4)

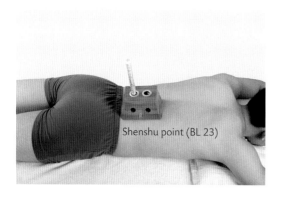

Shenshu point (BL 23)

Moxibustion with moxa stick roll holder: Moxibustion is applied to the Shenshu point and then the Guanyuan point. The person receiving moxibustion should take an appropriate posture. Place a moxa stick roll holder on the point for moxibustion, ignite a moxa roll and put it on the mesh, and then close the cover to perform moxibustion. Moxibustion lasts 20 to 30 minutes for each point, once every 2 to 3 days for a 1- to 3-month course of treatment with an interval of 3 to 5 days between two courses. This therapy is characterized by balanced distributed heat, which makes the person receiving moxibustion feel comfortable.

APPENDIX

INDEX

T

Taichong point   29, 35, 43–45, 52, 53, 64, 65, 75, 76, 82–84, 97, 101, 113, 124, 125

Taixi point   29, 72, 73, 85–89, 93, 94, 99, 100, 121–125, 132, 133

Taiyang point   29, 135–137

Taiyuan point   30, 103, 104

Tianshu point   21, 32, 35, 37–40, 90, 91, 129

Tiantu point   34, 35, 103, 104

Tianzhu point   58, 59

Tinggong point   21, 122–124

Tinghui point   122–124

Tongli point   107

Tongziliao point   51, 52

Touwei point   29

W

Waiguan point   27, 28, 52, 53

Weishang point   40, 41

Weishu point   32, 36, 38, 39, 82, 91, 92, 96, 102, 103, 129

X

Xiaguan point   48, 91, 92

Xiaochangshu point   91, 92

Xiawan point   39, 40

Xiaxi point   43, 44, 52, 53

Xingjian point   43, 44, 66, 68

Xinshu point   55, 85–88, 106, 107, 111, 112, 133, 134

Xuanji point   103, 104

Xuanzhong point   56, 61, 62

Xuehai point   52, 53, 61, 62, 66–68, 72, 93, 94

Y

yang   11, 12, 19, 22, 24, 49, 66, 76, 86, 88, 99, 101, 112, 113

yang qi   11, 112

Yangbai point   91, 92, 136, 137

Yangfu point   29

Yanglingquan point   56, 61, 62, 64, 65, 84, 113, 114, 123, 124

Yaoyangguan point   59–61, 86, 87, 117, 118, 130, 131

Yifeng point   91, 92, 122–124

yin   19, 24, 33, 72, 73, 86, 90, 99, 113, 139

Yinbai point   77, 78

Yingxiang point   93, 94, 96

Yinjiao point   72, 75

Yinlian point   72, 75, 76

Yinlingquan point   37, 38, 68, 75, 76, 83, 85–87, 90, 91

Yintang point   21, 48, 91, 92, 96

Yongquan point   33, 34, 41, 42, 44, 45, 49, 101, 132, 133

Yuyao point   51, 52

Z

Zhangmen point   36, 53, 54, 114, 115

Zhigou point   32

Zhishi point   117, 118, 124, 125

Zhongfu point   53, 54

Zhongji point   66–68, 71, 72, 75–78, 83, 84, 86, 87, 89, 124, 125

Zhonglushu point   72

Zhongwan point   11, 33–36, 38–41, 82, 90, 91, 99, 100, 108, 114–116, 129, 130

Zhongzhu point   123, 124

Zigong point   67, 68, 75, 76, 124, 125

Zusanli point   11, 25, 32–43, 47, 55, 61, 64, 65, 67–70, 73, 75–78, 82, 89–91, 93, 94, 99, 100, 107–109, 111–113, 124, 125, 127, 128, 130, 131, 135, 139